10]

A. Aduboffour
17/5/2013

Sex and Romance During Pregnancy and After the Birth

What expectant couples need to know

Adelaide E Aduboffour

authorHOUSE®

AuthorHouse™ UK Ltd.
500 Avebury Boulevard
Central Milton Keynes, MK9 2BE
www.authorhouse.co.uk
Phone: 08001974150

First published by AuthorHouse 7/28/2010

ISBN: 978-1-4520-2274-1 (sc)

This book is printed on acid-free paper.

Contents

Acknowledgements

Very special thanks go to Joe, my dearest husband, and my two wonderful daughters, Tracy and Wilma, for their support and understanding.

I would like to thank all the couples who provided information and shared their experiences. Special thanks to Rajesh and Preetha Ramkumar, Ishara and Daniel Sule, Leon and Lucy Peacock for their invaluable contribution.

My deepest appreciation goes to Helen Boateng, Supervisor of Midwives; Sally Seaman, Community Midwife; Beverley Bogle, Lecturer in Midwifery and Women's Health Studies, King's College, for their continuous support and professional advice. I would also like to thank my colleagues and friends who supported and motivated me, especially Sinead Burns, Kimberley Solomon and Henrietta Nheta.

Many thanks to Owen Williams (www.owen.arts.co.uk) for the illustrations and Carrie Bartkowiack for her educational poem about pregnant women. A special word of thanks to 123RF images and ICEA, for their permission to reproduce their images.

I am grateful to Claire Gillman, Martin Ouvry and Tara Foss for their editorial assistance.

Foreword

Rarely does one get the opportunity to write a foreword for a book about sex and romance in pregnancy and childbirth!

This is a book for any woman who is pregnant, has been pregnant, or who is contemplating pregnancy, and wondering about the impact this may have on her relationship with her husband or partner. For most, pregnancy is the culmination of a very close relationship.

Whilst this subject may have been discussed in whispers with a close female friend, at last we have a delightfully clear and frank explanation of many of the issues that affect women going through the childbirth process. I am glad that I will be able to refer friends, family and clients to this knowledgeable and factual text.

My congratulations to Adelaide for being brave enough to bring all of the information together in one compelling read!

Fiona Ghalustians
    Senior Midwife, Supervisor of Midwives
    West Middlesex Hospital
    London

Preface

Promoting wellbeing for pregnant women and their families has always been my passion. After working as a nurse in London for four years, I enrolled at Thames Valley University, London, where I obtained a degree in midwifery. I have been practising midwifery in the NHS since 2005.

With my knowledge of the physical and psychological changes that occur in women's bodies during pregnancy, I realised that complementary therapy could be beneficial to them. I acquired a Level 3 Diploma in Holistic Massage (awarded by the International Therapy Examination Council) at St Mary's College, London. I then went on to specialise in pregnancy and baby massage.

Women use my massage services for a variety of reasons; for example, to relieve backaches, sciatica and fatigue and to promote relaxation. For others it is simply to have human contact and talk about any issues they cannot (or will not) discuss at their antenatal appointments or with their midwife. The trust I built with these women allowed them to open up to me and ask questions and voice concerns about sex and childbirth. The impression I got from most women (and their partners) confirmed that information about sex during pregnancy is scant or is not discussed by midwives, obstetricians or GPs. The most common concern for parents-to-be is whether the penis will hurt the unborn baby or if sex can cause a miscarriage. Some of the mums were worried about resuming sex after delivery, for a variety of reasons.

After childbirth, an important minority of women have complications such as urinary incontinence; some have perineal tears after delivery which are not sutured or are badly sutured. Poor after-care of perineal wounds can cause severe pain, wound-infection and gaping. Some women suffer in silence before reporting these issues because they feel embarrassed to talk about it. Some may even think what they are experiencing is normal with childbirth. It's not. These problems can lead to sexual dysfunction, which inevitably affects the couple's sex life. Lack of education in this area can have an enormous psychological and physical impact on relationships, and, in some cases, result in the breakdown of the relationship.

It was because of these concerns that I began to explore this important topic: sex in relation to pregnancy and childbirth. Over the course of 18 months, I spoke to parents and expectant couples from different ethnic, socio-cultural and educational backgrounds about their experiences. Their responses were varied and interesting. I also had informal discussions with some midwives and obstetricians to gain their views. I researched the available literature – professional articles and books, and information intended for couples. My own observations whilst caring for couples in labour were also very helpful.

I wrote this book because the information I found in all those sources was worth putting together in one place to share with couples, midwifery students and healthcare professionals. Some of my colleagues, friends and clients also encouraged me to write it. Stella*, a mum of two, said, "I found information on sex and childbirth in other pregnancy books and on the internet, but it is more reassuring to hear it from your midwife."

As a midwife, a wife and a mother of two, I believe in not only promoting the physical wellbeing of couples, but also the emotional and psychological wellbeing in which sex, love and affection play a major role. I've aimed this book at pregnant women, but the information included is just as valuable and important to men, so please share these pages with your partner. After you read this book, I hope you will have a better understanding of how childbirth affects your sexual life, and how you and your partner can work together, with understanding, to make the entire experience enjoyable.

*All names in this book have been changed to protect contributors' privacy.

Introduction

Pregnancy and childbirth is a life-changing experience for you and your partner. There are many physical and emotional changes that occur which affect your relationship and sex life. This book explores the physical and psychological changes during pregnancy, and how they may affect sex and relationships. The practical experiences of real couples will also be shared throughout, as will tips to help you make the most of your love life during this life-changing time. Different sexual positions will be suggested to make sex easier as the "bump" grows bigger. I discuss pregnancy complications, and why you need to be gentle or refrain from sex when those complications arise. Even when sexual intercourse is avoided by choice or by medical advice, this book explores how you and your partner can stay close to each other to maintain your intimacy.

I have also gathered together some attitudes, myths, cultural and religious beliefs surrounding sex and childbirth for you to read about. You may be surprised by some of them, or they may be very familiar. Either way, the chapter is designed to help you understand this time of life across the world.

At any point in life, people can experience changes in their sex drives. These changes are even more common during pregnancy and after birth. For many couples, the new experience brings togetherness and unbridled fondness. The intimacy may improve your sex life and make your relationship stronger. However, a sexual slowdown is also fine: it is perfectly normal to lose interest in sex during pregnancy and the postnatal period until you are physically and psychologically ready.

During the second trimester, when nausea, fatigue and fears of miscarriage are usually over, you may discover that you are more interested in sex. At the same time, your partner may not want to have sex as often as he did before the pregnancy. While some women joke that men are simple creatures, this is far from the truth; your pregnancy can affect his sex drive and he might not know how to talk about it with you. He might be scared of hurting the unborn baby. He might worry that you will feel angry if he finds you less sexually alluring during the last few months of your pregnancy. It is during this time especially that communication must be open, honest and caring. This book will help you learn how to make that happen.

On the other hand, some women may also use pregnancy as an excuse to turn their partners away, saying that they aren't in the mood to have sex. This is common with women whose partners have a high sex drive. You may be experiencing physical discomfort, especially towards the end of your pregnancy. As your "bump" grows, you may find lovemaking uncomfortable. Your desire for sex may decrease. Your partner might feel neglected, rejected and unloved if you do not communicate with him.

Both men and women have expressed their frustration about missing sex with their partners. In the past, some of my clients have used me as an advocate to explain to their spouse how they feel when sex is becoming more frequent than they can bear, or vice versa.

Isha and Ali had been married for one year and were expecting their first baby. Ali wanted to have sex almost every day. Isha said she could not cope with the pace. She was having constant lower abdominal pain and she couldn't figure out whether it was the pregnancy or the regular intercourse. She couldn't tell Ali how she felt. Instead, she used me, her midwife, as an advocate when she attended her first antenatal booking appointment. I advised them to discuss the issue honestly and come to a reasonable compromise.

Ali felt Isha could have opened up and told him at home. He did not realise it was too much for her. He thought he was performing his marital duties to please his wife. But pleasing a woman and meeting her sexual needs is not all about the frequency of sex: increased intimacy such as confiding in each other, cuddling, and romantic gestures like lighting candles at dinner, or massaging each other, can please her as well.

Ali's compromise was light-hearted: "Isha, how about alternate days if you cannot cope with it every day?" But lovemaking should be spontaneous. Drawing a timetable for sex can kill the excitement and turn it into a chore instead of pleasure. You should have sex when you are ready and comfortable.

Clearly it is important for you to be honest and practical about discussing sex with your partner. You need to have open discussions about how you feel to defuse any frustration. Regardless of your normal sex drive, this is a time when you need to be intimate and share a lot of love and affection with your partner.

The most common questions raised by couples are: Is it safe to have sex? Will sex hurt my unborn child or cause discomfort to my partner? What is the best position to have sex as the "bump" grows? Will sex start off my labour? When is the best time to resume sex after the birth of the baby? While all these questions are playing on your mind, who should you go to for answers and reassurance?

Sex may not be easy to discuss with friends and family, unless you have a special relationship with them whereby you can discuss anything and everything. Some new parents said they read about it on the internet or spoke to friends about it. Others said it was briefly mentioned at the antenatal classes. However, although sexuality and sex are more openly discussed today on television, through the internet and in schools, most people still find it very difficult or embarrassing to discuss sex during pregnancy with the midwife or healthcare professional. These feelings may be influenced by how we were brought up culturally and socially. As we grew to adolescence, most of our parents found it embarrassing to discuss sex and puberty with us. It is all hush-hush! Everything is kept under wraps. People who talk openly about sex may be perceived as rude or uncultured. As a result of these perceptions, some couples may find it difficult or uncomfortable to open up to each other.

The subject of sex during pregnancy can be difficult for midwives and doctors to explore with couples because it is private. As a couple, you may also feel uncomfortable or embarrassed to talk about an intimate topic like sex to an outsider, especially if you are meeting them for the first time. Some midwives only raise the topic when they recommend it as a natural way of inducing labour at the end of your pregnancy. Your midwife may briefly discuss sex in relation to family planning after you've had your baby, but she may not explore how you feel about resuming sex following the birth, especially if you had an instrumental delivery, a tear, or an episiotomy (an incision made at the perineum by the midwife or the doctor to aid the delivery of your baby).

This reminds me of when I was assisting a doctor one night in theatre to repair an episiotomy for a first-time mum. Anka had an instrumental delivery of a 9lb 12oz baby boy. I noticed that Anka and her husband Philippe were curious and asking the doctor questions like: How long will it take for the wound to heal? Will the stitches need to be removed? How many stitches did she have? I could see the anxiety in Philipe's face. He even stretched his neck to see if the doctor had done a "good job". I guessed they wanted to know about the impact on their sex life, but they were obviously not going to ask the question "in public" – in the presence of the other staff. The doctor explained everything to them after the procedure, and gave them advice on pain relief, how to avoid constipation and prevent infection, and when to start pelvic floor exercises. The only thing the doctor did not mention was sex; maybe she didn't know how to address the subject in front of other people in the room. I also knew that she was not going to get the chance to talk to them about it in private. I went close to them and whispered to them, "We will talk about sex later." They both burst into laughter and were keen to have that conversation with me at the appropriate time. I went to have a chat with them in the postnatal ward, and they found the information very helpful.

CHAPTER I

Understanding the changes of your body during pregnancy

As you will no doubt know, during pregnancy your body undergoes many changes caused by pregnancy hormones. Some of the common minor problems that you may experience are nausea, vomiting, excessive salivation, dizziness, tiredness, excessive vaginal discharge, breast tenderness, and a feeling of anxiety during the first 12 weeks. You may be irritable and experience mood swings. When you feel unwell, the last thing on your mind is sex and, as discussed in the Introduction, your sexual desire may fluctuate throughout the pregnancy. But do not be surprised if other women tell you that they sailed through their pregnancy without suffering from any of these minor ailments.

> *Yasmin's experience*
>
> *When I was expecting Lucinda, my first daughter, I kept looking forward to when the pregnancy symptoms would start, but they never did. I was active throughout my pregnancy. I enjoyed sex better, especially during the second trimester. My libido was heightened, which made me chase my husband around for more sex. I did not have to worry about falling pregnant or using contraception, which made me more relaxed. I found it very exciting changing to different positions to adapt to the growing bump, and my husband just went with the flow.*

After the first three months, most women feel energised as the early pregnancy symptoms begin to settle. You will begin to relax into your new role as mum-to-be. Increased blood flow to the genital area and breast enlargement can make you more sexually aroused. Your partner will also enjoy sex because of the warmth in your vagina due to the increased blood flow.

Physical changes

Nausea and vomiting

You may experience nausea and vomiting during the first few weeks of pregnancy. Even though it is known as morning sickness, it can occur any time of the day, but it is very common in the mornings when you brush your teeth. During early pregnancy you may also struggle to tolerate strong smells of perfume, body lotions or spicy foods. There are several things you can do to at least minimise the sickness:

- Try to eat a healthy, well-balanced diet;
- Cut down on fatty food and deep fried food;
- Increase your fruit and vegetable intake;
- Just eat what you can tolerate in small amounts;
- Drink plenty of fluids;
- Some women say they find ginger (in capsules, as a tea or in foods) helpful as it can help reduce the nausea;
- Keep the romance alive. Let your partner bring toast or biscuits to you in bed if you feel unwell.

You may also have extreme cravings, sometimes for non-food substances such as coal, soap, toothpaste, chalk, or wall paint. This is known as *pica*, the Latin word for magpie, a bird known to eat almost anything. These cravings are thought to arise from vitamin and mineral deficiencies, so it is vital to watch what you eat and get proper nutrition. Also, cravings for non-nutritional substances can compromise your health and that of your unborn baby, and should be avoided.

Get your partner involved in planning your meals to figure out what works for you so that you get the nutrition you need. He will also feel involved in the process and feel useful. Working together as a team will make you feel supported and will encourage you to eat even if you have poor appetite. It also reduces your workload at a time when you need more rest.

Vomiting can cause dehydration and weakness, so you need to drink plenty of fluids to rehydrate. Tell your doctor or midwife if it gets worse. Dehydration can also lead to bad breath, so you will still need to brush your teeth (even if it makes you nauseous). If you are dehydrated your lips will get dry and crack easily, so apply lip balm or lipstick to keep them moist. Besides, good oral hygiene will make you feel more like kissing.

Tender breasts

During pregnancy, your breasts may feel tender and heavy, similar to when you are about to have your period. The breast increases in size, it feels full and firm. The enlargement of the breasts can make you feel sexually aroused and enhance sex for you and your partner. Some women, however, feel very uncomfortable when their breasts are touched during lovemaking. If you experience any discomfort, you should tell your partner to be gentle. Do not suffer in pain for fear of offending him.

Tips for partners

Make sure she feels comfortable when you touch her breast. You need to be gentle and sensitive. Look at her facial expression and notice how she responds to your touch. Talk to her and find out if she is enjoying it. There will be no pleasure for her if she experiences pain or discomfort.

Did you know?

Towards the end of pregnancy the breast starts to secrete colostrum, a precursor of breast milk. Your partner may taste some breast milk if he sucks on your nipples during lovemaking.

Skin changes

Most women are self-conscious of the changes to their skin, such as stretch marks, and these may hinder their desire for sex. You may feel unattractive and believe your partner feels the same way about you. The good news is, not all the skin changes are negative. Your face becomes dewy, because the pregnancy hormones cause increased secretions from the oil glands. Your blood volume increases by almost 50 per cent, which causes your cheeks to take on a reddish blush. As a result, you glow and look beautiful.

On the negative side, stretch marks may occur as your size increases. Stretching occurs in the collagen layer of your skin, particularly over the breasts, tummy and thighs. Some women get them, some don't; it depends on your skin type. The area of maximum stretch changes to glistening, silvery white lines, which are less noticeable some months after birth. It is doubtful if creams or oils help to prevent stretch marks, but generally there is no harm in using the oils and creams as long as they are natural products and contain no harsh chemicals. They will help to moisturise your skin and it can feel very good if your partner helps you to apply them.

From the third month until birth, some degree of skin darkening is observed in the majority of pregnant women. This is more obvious in black women. You may also notice a dark line running over your tummy, known as the linea nigra. You may develop pigmentation on the face; this affects at least half of pregnant women. It is called chloasma or melasma, and is also known as "the mask of pregnancy". You can apply make-up to hide it.

Itchy skin is not common, but if it occurs it can be distressing. It may be due to dry skin or stretching of the skin. In this case, applying body lotion can help moisturize the skin to stop the itching. If it continues, you need to tell your midwife or doctor for medication to sooth the itching. A blood test may be required to rule out obstetric cholestasis (a liver condition that develops in pregnancy; its cause is unknown).

Varicose veins / piles

During pregnancy, high levels of the hormone progesterone can cause relaxation of the muscles around the veins, causing varicose veins. If you already have this condition, it may become worse. Varicose veins usually appear in the thighs and legs. If they appear in the anal area, they are called haemorrhoids, or piles, and can itch and bleed. They are often caused by straining to open your bowels when you are constipated. Varicose veins on the vulva can also be very painful. Sex will not appeal to you if you are in pain or uncomfortable. You can apply a cold or warm flannel to ease the discomfort, and see your midwife or doctor if it gets worse.

Tina's story

Tina was expecting her second baby when she noticed varicose veins on her vulva. She did not have varicose veins at all during her first pregnancy. She said, "It was strange to me. I thought varicose veins only appear on the legs and thighs. I didn't know that they can actually appear on your 'fanny' [vulva]." She added, "I felt embarrassed to discuss it with my husband or my midwife. Pete could not understand why I was not interested in having sex. I was about 26 weeks pregnant when he booked a short weekend break in France for the two of us. He was hoping that the change of environment would relax me and bring back my desire for sex. I found sex off-putting because it was uncomfortable and awkward. I enjoyed the weekend break but still could not make love. I had to gather courage and tell him about the discomfort. He was very understanding and caring."

Vaginal discharge

It is normal for you to have more than your usual vaginal discharge during pregnancy. It is a colourless and non-irritating discharge called leucorrhoea. Some couples find sex more enjoyable with the increased lubrication; others may not find it pleasurable if the excessive lubrication reduces the friction of the penis in the vagina. It is not normal if the discharge causes itching, is thick, bloodstained, or has an offensive odour. These symptoms may be due to cervical erosion, Candida (commonly known as thrush, with a white, curdled discharge), or a sexually transmitted infection, such as Chlamydia.

What to do if you have these symptoms:

- See the midwife or the doctor to rule out infection;
- Avoid washing out the vagina with water or other mixture of fluids (douching), since it can cause irritation in the vagina and the vulva;
- Wash frequently with water;
- Wear loose cotton underwear and panty liner;
- In the case of infection, your doctor will prescribe treatment;
- Avoid sex until the infection is cleared. Your partner will also need to see a doctor for treatment;
- You may be referred to a sexual health clinic.

Passing urine frequently

This occurs during the first 12 weeks of pregnancy as a result of the pressure of the growing womb on your bladder. The pressure is eased after three months, when your womb moves upwards, away from the bladder. During late pregnancy, the pressure of the baby's head presses on your bladder and it recurs. You will make frequent trips to the toilet, and it can disturb your sleep during the night. If you normally make love in the middle of the night, you may be tired and may struggle to keep awake for sex, so try morning sex instead.

If the frequency of passing urine is accompanied by pain and a burning sensation, fever or backache, it may be a urinary tract infection (UTI). If you experience signs of a UTI, try to:

- *Drink plenty of clear fluids (water, fruit juice);*
- *Contact your doctor for a urine test and treatment;*
- *Wash the vulva area frequently with water to avoid odour;*
- *When you wipe yourself after passing urine or opening your bowels, remember to wipe yourself from front to back. If you do the opposite, you may introduce infection from your back passage (anus) to the urine passage (urinary tract).*

Body pains and aches

As your baby grows, you may adopt a different posture to balance the weight. Your back hollows and your bump pushes forward, causing backache. You are thrown off balance by your growing bump, and your spine compensates to support you. Relaxation of the ligament supporting the pelvic bone can also be blamed for backache. Backache that comes and goes in a pattern may signify the onset of labour. Try to have plenty of rest and relax. Gentle massage and aromatherapy are usually beneficial. Sexual intimacy can reduce stress. As long as you are comfortable, there is no reason why you cannot indulge in lovemaking. Remember that making love should be pleasurable, not painful. If you find a particular position uncomfortable, tell your partner and try a different one.

Sleeplessness

Sleeplessness is very common in late pregnancy and is usually due to:

- The discomfort of your baby's movement;
- Your muscles stretching;
- Passing urine frequently;
- Difficulty in finding a comfortable position.

Sleeplessness and exhaustion may make you irritable; few people fancy sex when they are in that state. Most women feel anxious as labour draws closer. Clear information about labour and your options for pain relief will help ease the anxiety. You may find lovemaking a good way to release tension, or you may go off it completely. Sharing your feelings as a couple will help.

To help induce sleep or have better, more restful sleep, try the following:

- Use comfortable pillows. You may find you like different pillows at different stages of pregnancy. Try a full-body pillow or a wedge-shaped pillow for extra comfort;
- Sleep on a firm mattress for support and comfort;
- Keep the bedroom at a comfortable temperature;
- Try a glass of warm milk before bed;
- Dim the lights, play relaxing music, massage each other.

The growing bump / weight gain

Your bump will begin to show at around 24 weeks, and you will be visibly pregnant. You may experience rib pain because the baby is pressing upwards against the ribcage. The rapid weight gain starts about now. Your heart and lungs will double up their work rate, so this is not the time to diet; instead, eat a variety of fresh, unprocessed and nutritious foods.

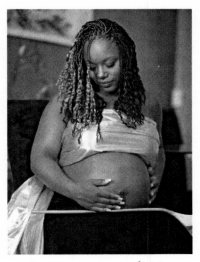

A pregnant woman admiring her new shape.

You will not be able to reach your feet easily when showering or to apply body lotion. Shaving the pubic area will become more difficult as the bump grows bigger. Your partner can help you in the shower to wash your feet, with shaving and with trimming your nails. Helping you with little things like these can enhance intimacy.

Some women feel sexy and attractive about their new body. For such women, the bump reinforces or enhances their femininity; other women may feel shapeless and clumsy. Your pregnancy shape is something you should be proud of and enjoy. You will be pleased to know that most men find the pregnant body extremely sensuous, attractive and sexy

Maintain good personal hygiene

Dr Barbara De Angelis, the author of *Secrets About Men Every Woman Should Know*, revealed that men get turned off by poor personal care and hygiene – as much as we get turned off by theirs. Among the long list were:

- Bad breath;
- Wearing baggy dresses;
- Unpleasant vaginal smell;
- Body odour;
- Unkempt hair;
- Unshaved under arms and legs (although some cultures may find this attractive).

Your natural body and vaginal odour can turn your partner on during lovemaking. However, increased vaginal discharge, passing urine frequently and sweat can cause unpleasant odours. You are more prone to infections such as thrush and urinary tract infection during pregnancy. Vomiting can cause dehydration, which will increase the ketone level in your blood, which can cause bad breath. Your partner may not find it easy to tell you that you have bad breath or body odour for fear that he might hurt your feelings or embarrass you. He may simply avoid kissing you or having sex with you. If you notice these issues, it is likely he has too. Let him know that many of these issues will pass, but in the meantime, try the following to help you feel better:

1. Have a shower or bath regularly.
2. Wash your vulva by parting the labia (the folds) and gently wash with mild soap and water. Stop using soap if it causes irritation.

3. Wear a panty liner and change it frequently.
4. You can help prevent thrush by wearing loose cotton underwear, but if you get it, contact the doctor or your midwife for treatment and avoid sex until the infection is cleared.
5. Frequent mouth-care is essential to feel refreshed. Drink plenty of fluids to prevent dehydration and bad breath.

Feel good and look sexy

It can be difficult to get dressed every day when you feel sick, clumsy and heavy. But a little effort to stay active can make you feel energised or perhaps a bit like your pre-pregnancy self. Looking good reflects how you feel inside, and it is a common belief that how you feel reflects the way you look. Staying active and getting ready for the day will help you feel rejuvenated, attractive and sensual. Good make-up is one of the little secrets that can make you feel pretty and in control, especially when you feel you've lost control of your body. Getting a manicure and pedicure, a pregnancy massage or a specialist spa treatment, can lift your spirit and boost your self-esteem.

Comfort is usually the first thing that comes to mind when you think of maternity wear. You can still wear clothes that offer comfort, quality and flattering styles. These days, there are many choices for pregnant women who want to stay fashionable. There are trousers and jeans with waistbands that adjust as your shape changes. More and more maternity dresses and tops hug your form to show off your beautiful bump.

Don't forget that your bra size will increase too. Wear supportive bras; if you normally wear an underwire bra, you may feel more comfortable wearing wireless bras during your pregnancy. Pregnancy should not stop you from wearing pretty knickers and fancy bras. Experiment with colours and shapes and you will be surprised how sexy you will feel. At this time, stop wearing high-heel shoes because they can aggravate a backache or cause you to become unbalanced. Flat shoes (especially ones you don't have to tie) are recommended during your pregnancy.

Psychological changes

Having a baby means a huge emotional change for you and your partner. Most people are happy and excited when they learn that there is a new baby on the way, but you and your partner may have mixed feelings about becoming parents. Both of you may be bombarded with information from health professionals, pregnancy books, friends and family. You will hear about other people's experiences – both positive and negative. Some people around you may react differently to the news, depending on the circumstances that led to the pregnancy. The following are just some of the most common emotional changes during pregnancy.

Moods

Mood changes are a reflection of the change in hormonal secretions. You may experience extremes of emotion: you may get more easily upset and tearful about little things, and the next moment feel happy. As the due date gets closer, you will have mixed feelings. You will look forward to meeting your baby, and at the same time be anxious that all goes well with the birth. Most couples hear about different birth experiences from other couples, and it's normal that the negative experiences cause some anxiety. Most women are worried about how they will cope with the labour pains. The majority are also worried about opening their bowels during the birth. These thoughts, though normal, can make you lose interest in lovemaking as the expected date of delivery draws closer.

Remember that every birth experience is different. Attending antenatal classes or reading the pregnancy books together can give you and your partner correct and clear information. However, some people don't like too much information. They end up being stressed by it. They think everything they read will happen to them or their baby. Talk to your midwife or doctor if you have any concerns. Your plan of care in labour should be discussed with you. Don't be afraid to ask for further explanation if things are not clear. It may be difficult to take everything on board when you are in pain, so instead rely on your partner, birth coach, midwife or doctors to help you understand.

Body image and pregnancy

Apart from your growing bump and weight gain, some of your features may become exaggerated. While some women are not bothered and understand that it is natural for their body to undergo such changes, others feel unattractive and unsexy. Your nose and lips may get thicker; your clitoris and labia can become more prominent. The good news is that the engorgement of your clitoris and labia can heighten your sexual response and increase sexual pleasure for you and your partner.

Some women may find it very difficult to expose their naked pregnant body in front of their lover. They may prefer to make love with the lights turned off. Reassurance from your partner is one key to this psychological issue. According to Dr Miriam Stoppard, the UK's favourite childcare expert, your image of yourself during pregnancy is important. Feeling proud of your increasing curves and your fertility should make you more positive about your condition and encourage you to take a general interest in looking good. You should feel confident and proud of your rounded body: think of it as reaffirmation of life.

Unplanned pregnancy

If you fall pregnant unexpectedly, in the beginning of a new relationship, or while in a struggling relationship, you may wonder if your partner will accept the pregnancy as you struggle to come to terms with it yourself. You may not even be in love with each other. Some women will consider terminating an unwanted pregnancy. If the man feels the pregnancy is being used to commit him to the relationship, this may lead to anger and tension, which is not the ideal recipe for happiness, let alone romance and lovemaking. On the other hand, some couples may be happy about the surprise of pregnancy, and it will have no negative effects on their relationship or sex life.

Birth defects

Every expectant couple hope that their baby will be healthy, and most babies are. However, a few babies do have problems, such as a cleft palate, spina bifida or Down's syndrome. If a couple is expecting a baby with congenital abnormalities, or has previous experience of a birth defect, they will be more anxious and stressed, which may mean their desire for sex is diminished. They may also be concerned that they may cause further damage to their unborn child if they engage in penetrative sex. (This isn't possible by the way. See Chapter 3).

Infertility, previous pregnancy and birth experience

Those who have experienced fertility problems, previous miscarriages, premature labour and delivery or previous stillbirth may be over-protective of the unborn baby. As much as they are excited, they will also be concerned that nothing should go wrong with the pregnancy. Reassurance from the healthcare professionals and caring words from your partner are important, so don't be embarrassed to ask for either.

Sex or no sex?

Anisa and Jokim had waited for six years after their marriage to conceive. When Anisa eventually fell pregnant naturally, she was excited. She said, "I didn't want to do anything silly like having sex to hurt my baby or start labour prematurely. We had a good sex life for six years, I'm sure I can do without sex for a few months for the sake of my baby."

Jokim said, "I sometimes had a strong desire to make love to Anisa. Initially, I felt pushed away and frustrated when she denied me sex. Eventually, I understood why she did not want to have penetrative sex. I tried to block sex out of my mind and engage in other activities, like going to the gym, swimming, taking her to the movies.

It was very difficult to start with, but I got used to it. I masturbated most of the time to relieve myself. We still kissed and cuddled each other. We both enjoyed it as the baby grew inside her. I touched her bump and felt the baby kicking; I felt I was bonding and communicating with the baby. I also felt reassured that both Anisa and baby were doing well. This wonderful experience drew Anisa and I closer emotionally."

At the other end of the spectrum, Sibo and Sifiso waited for 13 years before getting pregnant with their son. This created an even greater bond between them and they enjoyed sex throughout the pregnancy without worrying.

Changes that men may experience

Even though your partner is not physically carrying the pregnancy, he is expecting the baby, too. He experiences mixed emotions. He is happy for the good news that he is going to be a father, and at the same time feels anxious about how the whole experience is going to turn out. He may be confused and unsure of what his role is as an expectant dad. He may also feel under financial pressure to earn more money to care for you and the baby.

As you go through the physical changes, your partner can only imagine how you are feeling. He may feel you are vulnerable, and his natural instincts will make him want to protect you from any possible harm. He may be over-protective of you and the baby, and may be reluctant to have penetrative sex so as not to hurt you or the baby. He may feel worried and anxious when you feel unwell, or if there is any change from what he sees as "normal".

Some men may experience sympathetic pregnancy, also known as couvade syndrome. It comes from a French word meaning "to hatch" and it most often appears in the third month and again at delivery. It can mimic all the normal symptoms of pregnancy, such as morning sickness and mood changes.

Many men find it adventurous to witness their lover's changing body. Your partner may find your changing female body sensual, erotic and attractive. This may increase his desire to make love to you and he may feel rejected and unloved if you are never in the mood for sex. On another level, he may have a sense of guilt when he makes love to you. He feels responsible for all the changes you have to go through. This is why it is so important to have open and honest communication about your feelings toward sex during your pregnancy. There is no need for him to feel guilty when making love to you, and no reason for you to feel guilty for saying no. As long as you are well and comfortable, you *both* must enjoy sex.

There are a few men who may not find their partner's physical changes sexually appealing. This may lead to increased sexual problems, such as premature ejaculation, an erection failure or a problem maintaining an erection. His libido may be low and he may desire his pregnant partner less as a result. He may be concerned that he is making love to an "expectant mother with a baby growing inside her" instead of his lover. In most cases, these sexual problems are temporary and things may return to normal after delivery or once he overcomes his anxiety. If things don't resolve, seek help from a sexual counsellor.

Chris and Joan's story

Chris, 33, a lecturer, and Joan, 30, a manager, were told their chance of having a baby together was slim, because Joan was diagnosed with polycystic ovarian syndrome. After a romantic holiday in the Caribbean, they learned that Joan was pregnant. They were obviously very excited. Chris said, "From the moment I learned she was pregnant, I became over-protective, and as a result I didn't let her lift a cube of sugar. As the pregnancy grew bigger, I saw Joan's tummy and the baby inside her 'as delicate as an eggshell'. I found her pregnant body very attractive, but I was reluctant to have sex with her because I did not want to harm the baby or cause Joan any discomfort. I now realise that it is a mythical belief that having sex in pregnancy will harm the baby."

Work as a team

Some women will have the energy to work until the end of their pregnancy with no problems. Many women find that routine housework and other home duties are a good form of exercise and that their nesting instincts kick in. However, if you overdo it, you will feel tired, which will diminish your desire for sex. In some cultures it is the role of the woman to cook and do all the housework. The man is expected to be the main breadwinner even if the woman works as well. If you need him to help out around the house, he may find it difficult to adapt to this new type of supportive role, especially in the presence of friends and family. It may be deemed as weak to "assume the role" of the woman. It is rather the opposite. Supporting you with the housework and other chores shows how he loves and cares for you. There is nothing more romantic and loving than a supportive, understanding, caring partner. You are likely to be more responsive to sex if you feel loved and supported by him – and if you haven't spent all day cleaning the house.

In return, you need to show him that you appreciate his care and support. This will encourage him to do even more. As you begin to feel better and have fewer pregnancy symptoms, he may need you to make the first move for sex, especially if you were not interested in sex in the first few months. Even now, when you are not in the mood for sex, you can be intimate by cuddling to maintain closeness. You will both feel loved, and not emotionally or physically neglected. Talk to each other about your needs and concerns in an open and loving way. Working together will help you cope better and meet each other's sexual and romantic needs. If something does not feel physically or emotionally right for either of you, change it and try something else. Most men that I spoke to said they felt emotionally closer to their wives after doing some work around the house and appreciating the hard work she does.

I find the following poem, written by Carrie Bartkowiack, empowering for pregnant women. I hope reading it will make you feel more confident and sexy about your changing body.

Sensual Pregnancy

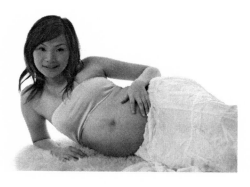

"And as his seed sprang in her, his soul sprang towards her too, in the creative act that is far more than procreative."
- D.H. Lawrence, Lady Chatterley's Lover

I loved being pregnant! I felt sexy and sensual, busty and beautiful. And every time I gazed upon my expanding belly I was reminded of that glorious act of love that had led to my baby's conception.

*Strangely enough, however, pregnant women are often looked upon as asexual. Although the very fact that a woman is pregnant means that **she has had sex**, society tends to view her as anything but sexual. It's as if she is suddenly expected to stop being a lover and start being a mother – and a virginal one at that.*

The problem with this line of thinking is that first of all, it's no fun, and secondly, it's unhealthy both physically and psychologically. Having sex and feeling sexual are crucial to a woman's sense of well-being. Pregnant women need to know and be told how beautiful they are – because, in truth, they are. Pregnancy, birth, and breastfeeding are integral parts of a woman's sex life. Accepting this fact will make all of them more pleasurable.

Chapter 2

Pelvic floor exercises . . . and how they enhance your sex life

What is the pelvic floor?

The pelvic floor consists of layers of muscles which stretch like a hammock from the pubic bone in front to the bottom of the spine. In women there are three openings in the pelvic floor: the urethra, the vagina and the anus.

Why your pelvic floor muscles are important

- They help to support the womb, the bladder and the bowel in place.
- They provide automatic muscle control for passing urine and opening your bowels.
- They also play an important role during pregnancy and childbirth, in that they support the weight of the unborn child, and during the second stage of labour the pelvic

floor muscles help your baby to turn and move forward ready for the birth.

Female Pelvic floor muscles and related organs

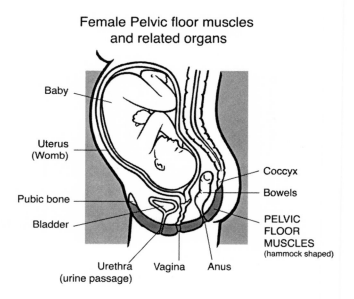

Baby

Uterus (Womb)

Pubic bone

Bladder

Coccyx

Bowels

PELVIC FLOOR MUSCLES (hammock shaped)

Urethra (urine passage)   Vagina   Anus

The pelvic floor muscles are kept firm and slightly tense to stop leakage of urine from the bladder and faeces from the bowel. When you open your bowels or pass urine, the muscles relax. Afterwards they tighten again to restore control. The pelvic floor muscles can become saggy or weak as a result of old age, lack of exercise, pregnancy and childbirth. If you have weak pelvic floor muscles you may leak urine when you laugh, cough or sneeze.

Why are pelvic floor exercises important?

Looking after your pelvic floor muscles is essential during pregnancy, following the birth, and throughout your life. Like any other muscle in the body, the more you exercise them, the stronger they become.

1. Pelvic floor exercises, also known as Kegel exercises, can strengthen the muscles to give support.

2. Pelvic floor exercises after birth will help you regain strength and function.

3. Women who sustain a natural tear or have a cut (episiotomy) during childbirth will also benefit if they do the pelvic floor exercises because the exercises cause increased blood-flow to the wound area. This, coupled with good nutrition and personal hygiene, will help the wound to heal quicker and reduce swelling and pain.

4. Longer-term toning up of the muscles will help your bladder and bowel control and improve or stop any leakage.

5. Doing Kegel exercises can also help prevent prolapse by making the pelvic floor muscles firmer and stronger.

6. Even if you had Caesarean section, you still need to do the pelvic floor exercise, as pregnancy may have weakened the pelvic floor muscles.

7. These exercises have the added benefit of giving you more control over the muscles you use when you have sex; and more control equals better sex.

Lucy's story

"I have two girls who were both born by Caesarean. The first one was an emergency, and the second one was planned. Any time I heard about pelvic floor exercise, I felt it was not for me because I had a Caesarean. Shortly after my second daughter was born, I noticed that my panty was frequently wet with urine. I did not have to sneeze or cough, it just happened. Initially, I did not want my husband to know; I felt embarrassed and uncomfortable to be intimate with him. It did not matter how frequently I washed myself, I still felt I smelt of urine. I took the bold step to speak to my GP about it. He referred me to the obstetric physiotherapist. Following the pelvic floor exercise programme, I noticed that the leakage had reduced after about four months. I do not leak any longer. I am more confident and my interest in sex has certainly improved. The exercise is now part of my daily routine. I usually do it at a red traffic light when I am driving!"

How to do pelvic floor exercises

Get yourself into any comfortable position. Imagine that you are trying to stop yourself from passing wind. Pull up the muscles surrounding your back passage, then pull up towards the front. The feeling is one of squeeze and lift, closing and drawing up the vagina and your anus. This is called pelvic floor contractions.

Hold tight as hard as you can for at least five seconds then relax. Repeat at least five times. These are called slow pull-ups. The fast pull-ups are when you pull the muscles up quickly and tightly, but release very quickly. This will help your muscles to react quickly when you laugh, sneeze, lift or cough. These exercises can be started within 24 hours of the birth of your baby. But do not do the exercises if you have a urinary catheter inserted.

Tips for pelvic floor exercises and beyond

1. During intercourse, try to squeeze the vagina tight around the penis and release. Try both the fast and the slow pull-ups and get feedback from your partner if the vaginal muscles are squeezing and releasing around his penis. Not only will you be doing the exercises, but you will both get pleasure.
2. Weight gain, which is normal in pregnancy, puts extra strain on your pelvic floor muscles. Exercise regularly and eat healthily.
3. Link the pelvic floor exercise to something you do often – for example, when you are talking on the phone, or when you are watching TV.
4. Drink plenty of water. Urinate only when you feel the urge to do so. Do not try to "hold on" to a full bladder for too long.

How do pelvic floor exercises help you to enjoy sex?

A strong pelvic floor muscle can greatly improve your sexual arousal, sexual response, the level of sensation you feel during lovemaking, and your ability to reach orgasm. The pelvic floor muscles are directly responsible for the amount of sensation women feel during sex. The ability to grip the penis with the vagina depends on how strong the muscles are. Pelvic floor exercises improve the muscle tone. They also make the muscles stronger, which improves sensation during sex.

Pelvic floor exercises also improve circulation, and this is very important for the smaller muscles of the pelvic floor. These muscles are responsible for engorging the clitoris when you are aroused. Rhythmic contractions of the pelvic floor help with arousal and, for most women, the ability to achieve orgasm. Many women testify that they are able to reach orgasm and enjoy sex better following frequent pelvic floor exercises.

Do men need to do pelvic floor exercises?

Men have the same pelvic floor as women. The only difference with men is that they have two openings, the anus and the urethra. Men can develop a weak bladder, sometimes following treatment for enlarged prostrate. Some men also experience premature ejaculation during sex, and this may be due to a weak pelvic floor. Pelvic floor exercises will make the muscles firmer and help improve his sex life.

Perineal massage during pregnancy

What is the perineum?

The perineum is the area of skin between the entrance to the vagina and the anal passage. During childbirth, the perineal tissues need to stretch to allow your baby to pass through the birth canal. Perineal massage during pregnancy helps to reduce the risk of perineal tears during childbirth.

Perineal trauma during childbirth

All women desire to give birth without perineal tears, cuts or stitches. Perineal tearing is a common occurrence during childbirth, and estimates suggest that over 85 per cent of women will sustain some degree of tearing during a vaginal birth. There are factors that can cause perineal tears regardless of perineal massage, such as instrumental delivery, anaemia, malnutrition and the integrity of your skin. To prevent a substantial tear, midwives or doctors may cut into the tissue to give the baby more room, a procedure called an episiotomy. It is possible to tear even if you have an episiotomy. The reduction in the use of routine episiotomy means that the majority of tears occur naturally. Tears are more common in women having their first vaginal birth, and range from small nicks and abrasions to deep lacerations affecting several pelvic floor muscles.

Classifications of tears:

- *First-degree tear is superficial and does not involve any muscles; it involves the skin of the perineum and the tissue around opening of the vagina or the outermost layer of the vagina itself. They usually heal quickly and cause little or no discomfort, and usually do not require stitches.*
- *Second-degree tear involves perineal skin and vaginal tissues, and goes deeper into muscles underneath. It requires stitches under local anaesthetic.*

> • *Third- and fourth-degree tears are rare. They involve the vaginal perineal skin, vaginal tissue and perineal muscles that extend into the anal sphincter (the muscle that surrounds your anus). A fourth-degree tear goes through the anal sphincter and the tissue underneath it. These tears need to be repaired layer by layer. They will cause you some discomfort and will usually take a few weeks to heal. The stitches dissolve on their own during the healing period. You will be given painkillers. Antibiotics are usually given in the case of third- or fourth-degree tear to reduce the risk of infection.*

What are the benefits of antenatal perineal massage?

Research shows that perineal massage during the last month of pregnancy enables the perineal tissue to expand more easily during birth, hence minimising your chances of tearing. Some researchers identify that the effect is clear for women who have not given birth vaginally before, and less clear for women who have. This may be due to the fact that those who have had a vaginal birth before had their perineum stretched when they had their first child. In that case, the massage may not make a significant difference.

1. The massage will enable you to familiarise yourself with the feeling of stretching and the pressure that occurs during the birth. It is most intense when your baby's head is being born.

2. Massaging daily will encourage the blood supply to your perineum, which helps with healing after birth.

3. If your partner is receptive to the idea, the use of perineal massage can offer a secondary benefit, that of foreplay, which can add to the sensual and erotic experience.

4. Your partner can feel he is playing a useful role in preparing your body for childbirth.

When do you start?

You can start at 34 weeks and continue until the end of the pregnancy. It doesn't take long – you can do it once a day for five minutes, preferably at a time you feel relaxed.

Preparing for the massage

1. Make sure the environment is warm, private and comfortable.

2. Take a relaxing bath, and then sit in a comfortable position with your legs apart. If you are doing it yourself, you may need a mirror to enable you to see what you are doing.

3. Whoever is doing the massage should wash their hands with soap and water and ensure that their nails are cut short and are smooth.

4. Use natural massage oil, like jojoba, sweet almond, olive or wheat germ oil, or a water-based lubricant like K-Y Jelly.

How is it done?

1. Apply some oil on the outside of the vagina and a small amount in the vagina.

2. Guide your thumb into the vagina for about 2 inches. Massage the muscle in a U-shaped fashion several times. If your partner is doing the massage, he can use his index finger.

3. Exert pressure with your thumb downwards for several seconds and release the pressure. When exerting the pressure, you may feel a tingling sensation as well as stretching. Continue the U-shaped massage with downwards thumb exertion for five minutes. You will notice that this muscle is easily stretched after one to two weeks.

4. The massage should be gentle, and not abrasive or vigorous.

5. Do the massage together with your pelvic floor exercises as a routine, to increase tone and control of your pelvic floor muscles.

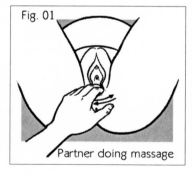

Fig. 01

Partner doing massage

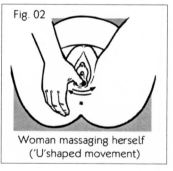

Fig. 02

Woman massaging herself
('U'shaped movement)

Feedback from some women

After speaking with several women, I learned that most of them found perineal massage helpful and did it regularly, while a few of the women found it unhelpful and uncomfortable.

Lizzy: "Initially I felt embarrassed to ask Nat, my partner, to do the perineal massage for me. I was not sure how he would feel about it. I thought it was gooey. I first encouraged him to read about it. To my surprise, he was comfortable with it. He said knowing that it would help prepare my perineum for childbirth made it even easier and he felt involved. After a few sessions both of us were more relaxed and it became a lot easier. I noticed I was more relaxed about the vaginal examinations performed by the midwives. My son was eight pounds and I had no tears. I feel the perineal massage was beneficial. It prepared me psychologically towards the second stage of labour. I will do it again with my second and subsequent pregnancies."

Grace: "I was keen to try anything and everything when I found out that I was pregnant with my first baby. I did lots of perineal massage. I could not reach easily towards the end of the pregnancy. I got my husband to help me. I still ended up with a second-degree tear. I don't think it made any difference in my case."

Laura: "*I found the perineal massage beneficial. As my bump got bigger, I could not reach easily, so I used a vibrator (switched off) dipped in grape seed oil. I also listened to my midwife. As my baby's head was halfway out (crowning), I began to really sting. I was tempted to scream and push so hard, to get it over and done with. My midwife was fantastic. She prepared me in advance to pant and do small pushes during crowning to let the perineum stretch gently, to minimise any tears. I only had small grazes in the vagina, with no perineal tears. I think the perineal massage definitely helped.*"

CHAPTER 3

Is it safe to have sex during pregnancy?

In the vast majority of cases it is safe to enjoy sex during pregnancy. The few exceptions to this are if you are bleeding, have a low-lying placenta (this will show on your 20-week scan), recurrent premature labour, or when your waters have broken. The bag of membranes and the amniotic fluid surrounding your baby, work like shock absorbers to protect the baby from any external trauma. Your baby is also protected by the muscles of the womb. The neck of the womb is closed and there is a plug of mucus which acts as a seal to prevent any infection from travelling to the baby. In normal low-risk pregnancy, sex may only start your labour at the very end of your pregnancy, when your body is ready to go into labour. Unless your cervix (neck of the womb) is "ripe", sex will not initiate labour (see Chapter 4).

Susan and Mark's story

Susan and Mark had been married for a year and were expecting their first baby. Susan said, "I did not want to have penetrative sex for the first three months because I was worried about miscarriage. Initially, Mark found it very difficult to cope with the idea, but he had to respect my choice and support me. We had a lot of cuddles, fondling and kisses. We watched movies, read pregnancy books together. We also massaged each other sometimes. Our love grew stronger because of the openness and the understanding we had for each other. I was very energetic from the fifth month and enjoyed sex."

Katherine and Glenn's experience

Katherine said, "When I was 16 weeks pregnant, I felt the baby kick while we were making love; I panicked and told Glenn to hurry up! When Glenn became aware of why he had been told to hurry up, he became scared and lost interest altogether. Glenn was worried that his penis had hurt the baby and that was why the baby kicked. From 16 weeks we avoided sex. When I got to 24 weeks, I had a strong desire to have sex again, but we were still worried. We read in a health magazine that it was safe. Thank God we found the truth and enjoyed sex again."

Just like Susan, many people are concerned that having penetrative sex will cause miscarriage, especially during the first three months. Like Katherine and Glenn, others fear it will harm their unborn baby. There is no evidence to suggest that sexual intercourse causes miscarriage or will harm the baby.

Some people feel that being pregnant is "medical" and may not want to have sex, especially if they are having a lot of tests done or are seeing doctors frequently. Certain conditions are not as severe or threatening as others. For example, some women can develop gestational diabetes, which can be controlled by diet or insulin. Others may suffer from hypertensive disorders, which may need medication or close monitoring. If you are diagnosed with any of these conditions, you may continue your sexual activities unless advised otherwise by your doctor.

Why the penis cannot hurt your baby

Regardless of what your partner thinks, the penis is not long enough to touch the baby during sex. It is normal for your baby to move during sexual intercourse – it does not mean your baby is being hurt.

- The vaginal wall is a long elastic canal;
- The neck of the womb is tilted backwards, and has a mucus plug blocking the entrance to protect the baby;
- The fore-waters in the membranes in front of the baby's head also serves as protection.

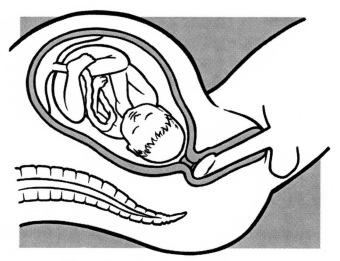

The Penis in the Vagina.

Baby Lucas was born with a swelling on his head. His parents thought that repeated intercourse had caused the swelling. They had sex just before Zahra went into labour that afternoon. I explained to them that the swelling was not caused by sex. It is a swelling of the scalp in a newborn, called caput succedaneum. This type of swelling is common and it occurs during prolonged labour or difficult delivery. After the waters are broken, the membranes no longer provide a protective cushion for the baby's head. The swelling is often brought on by pressure from the vaginal wall during head-first delivery. No treatment is necessary, as it usually resolves after a few days.

Benefits of sex during pregnancy

1. Aids physical and emotional bonding with your partner.
2. Prepares and tones your pelvic floor muscles, ready for childbirth.
3. You can enjoy a new sensual experience due to the hormonal changes.
4. No worries about falling pregnant, because you are already pregnant.
5. Helps to relieve stress.
6. Sex is a good mode of exercise.

Is the unborn baby aware when we have sex?

Your baby will not see you having sex and cannot remember it. Your baby is rather pacified by the gentle rocking motion of intercourse and the painless contracting uterus during orgasm.

When to avoid penetrative sex in pregnancy

Although most women can safely have sex throughout pregnancy, as I mentioned earlier in this chapter, there are unusual circumstances where your midwife or doctor will advise you to avoid penetrative sex during your pregnancy. You will be advised to abstain from sex during the first three months if you have had complications with previous pregnancies, such as premature labour, miscarriages or are experiencing cramping or bleeding.

Incompetent cervix

The term "incompetent cervix" (an inappropriate word to describe a woman's cervix) is widely used by medical professionals when the neck of your womb or cervix begins to open too soon. When this occurs, your baby could be born prematurely. If it is diagnosed in time, or if you had a previous experience of miscarriage, in the absence of contractions, the doctor can put a special stitch in the cervix to stop it from opening and leading to miscarriage.

Recurrent premature labour

If you have a history of premature labour, you will be advised by the obstetricians to refrain from sex. It is believed that orgasm may stimulate uterine contractions that may lead to premature labour. The avoidance of sexual activity may include no stimulation of the breasts as well.

Placenta praevia / low-lying placenta

Placenta praevia is when your placenta is situated at the lower part of your womb. The placenta could be positioned partially or completely over the opening of the neck of the womb. Placenta praevia is commonly diagnosed during your 20-week scan. A scan will be repeated to find out if the placenta is no longer low-lying. Although the placenta does not move (it stays attached at the same place), the growing uterus causes the relationship between the cervix and the placenta to change. In the majority of cases, it resolves, and you will be advised to carry on with your sexual activity as normal. In cases where the placenta praevia is not resolved, you will be offered additional ultrasound scans to monitor the pregnancy. If you have complete placenta praevia, you may be offered hospital admission for close monitoring. Your baby will be delivered by caesarean section as decided by your obstetrician. The management depends on each individual case.

You will then be advised by your doctor to refrain from penetrative sex. This is because sexual intercourse can cause bleeding, which can be life threatening for you and your baby. The doctor will recommend pelvic rest, which means:

- Avoid sex/orgasm;
- Avoid heavy lifting;
- Avoid any vigorous activities.

Normal Placenta

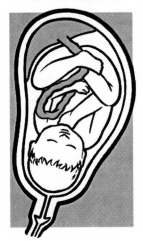 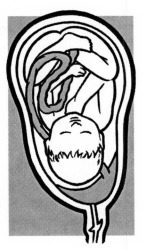

Placenta Praevia

Vaginal bleeding

In early pregnancy, you may experience light bleeding or spotting when your hormone levels are still low. Other causes of vaginal bleeding in pregnancy include miscarriage, ectopic pregnancy, infection, and placenta separating prematurely (placenta abruption). If you experience any bleeding, with or without pain, seek medical advice immediately, and obviously avoid having sex. In late pregnancy, a mucus discharge mixed with blood (known as a show) is an indication that your labour is about to start. It is normal, so do not panic.

Ruptured membranes (when your waters break)

When the water in front of the baby breaks, you will experience a gush, and your clothes will become very wet. It can be hard to tell if the water is leaking from behind the baby (hind water leak), because you may still feel a wet sensation. This may be confused with leaking urine due to the pressure of the baby's head on the bladder. The midwife will usually advise you to put a pad on for a while. If your waters have broken, the pad will be wet and not smell like urine. Amniotic fluid is normally cloudy white; if it is green, it means your baby has opened his bowels. This usually means your baby is not content and needs to be delivered sooner rather than later. You will be asked by the midwife to come into hospital for an assessment.

When the membranes are sealed, your baby is protected from any infections. Once the membranes are broken, it is advisable to refrain from sex, since infection can easily travel from the vagina to the baby and can make your baby unwell.

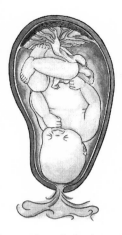

Baby in the womb with the fore waters broken

Can orgasm cause premature labour?

There is no evidence to suggest that orgasm can cause premature labour in a normal, low-risk pregnancy. After sex, you may experience that your bump is hard, but not painful, and this sensation will settle after a while.

I am expecting twins, can I have sex?

The over-stretching of the womb that occurs with twins is thought to increase the risk of premature labour. There is no evidence to support the theory that sex will cause premature labour. Just like women expecting single babies, you can equally enjoy sex in a gentle and sensible manner unless your doctor suggests otherwise.

Even though some people are well informed that sexual intercourse during normal pregnancy is safe, they may still choose not to have penetrative sex. As long as the two of you are comfortable and happy, you can find different ways of keeping close and intimate. For some couples, the conception of a wanted baby may heighten their sense of closeness and intimacy and increase tenderness during intercourse.

Intimacy beyond penetrative sex

According to relationship expert Dr Barbara De Angelis, there is a difference between having sex and making love. She says, "Having sex is the physical act of sharing pleasure with your partner. Making love is the emotional act of loving and adoring your partner." When penetrative sex is not possible for medical reasons or by choice, you can still express love to each other and show affection in many ways. Be creative and thoughtful – do things that will put a smile on your partner's face, and I bet he will respond by doing things to melt your heart. It feels good to appreciate each other. Some of the gestures that will go a long way are:

- Booking a surprise aromatherapy massage;
- Planning a romantic picnic;
- Buying roses or little presents for each other.

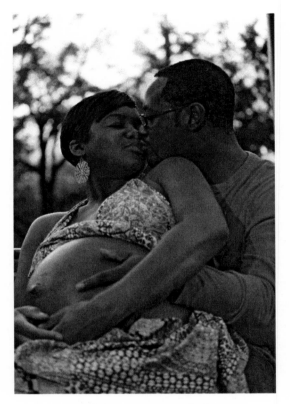

A couple keeping intimate by kissing

Keep the closeness by:

- Expressing your feelings to each other;
- Reminding each other of your love for one another;
- Cuddling, kissing;
- Massaging each other in a calm relaxing room (dim lights, romantic music and fragrance);
- Watching TV together in bed or on the sofa;
- Cutting or filing each other's nails;

- Doing something different and exciting from your usual routine;
- Arranging short weekends away from home.

Using sex toys, masturbation and oral sex

Pregnancy should not stop you from exploring other safe sexual practices if they are allowed by your religious and cultural beliefs. Masturbation, oral sex and the use of sex toys can be adventurous if you are trying them for the first time, or exciting if you know you enjoy them. Make sure your partner is comfortable with these options. If you desire to use sexual accessories like vibrators or "edibles" (gels or panties) for oral sex, you need to be more careful and sensible about it. If it is causing pain or discomfort, discuss it with your partner and stop and speak to the doctor or midwife.

Sex toys

If using sex toys is a normal part of your sex life, you can carry on as long as you have no complications in the pregnancy. Sex toys like vibrators are safe to use as long as you are gentle. However, their use inside the vagina may increase the risk of infection. To reduce the risk of infection, wash them thoroughly with soap and water before and after use and do not share. Avoid using any items in place of a sex toy (such as a bottle and similar objects) because, for example, the tip of the bottle may be cracked and cause injury in the vagina.

Some couples may use sex toys as a new adventure if they are uncomfortable having penetrative sex. If a couple is not having sex, one or the other partner may find that this helps to satisfy their sexual needs, taking pressure off the other partner to have sex. Your partner may, however, feel jealous if he finds out you're using a sex toy. He may wonder if you enjoy the sex toy more than him, especially if you stop approaching him for sex. You should explore this together to avoid any problems or misunderstandings.

Masturbation

Those who define sex as being equated solely with penis, vagina and sexual intercourse may find it more difficult to cope when penetrative sex is not an option. However, most people can and do enjoy self-masturbation or mutual masturbation. If penetrative sex is not an option, and if you are comfortable bringing up this topic with your partner, it can have excellent benefits for both of you.

Oral sex

It is safe to have oral sex in the absence of any genital infection if you and your partner are comfortable with it. Personal hygiene is essential if you are both to feel confident and comfortable. You can get a lot of pleasure from your partner stimulating your clitoris with his tongue. You can reach your climax without him penetrating the vagina with his penis. Equally, you can also perform oral sex on him. Most men enjoy receiving oral sex: apart from the pleasure it gives them, it can make them feel received and accepted. Avoid oral sex if you or your partner has cold sores or active genital herpes. Also avoid oral sex if you have thrush or any other vaginal infection until it is treated and cleared. For example, if your partner sucks your nipple straight after performing oral sex on you and you have thrush, he may introduce thrush to the nipples. He can also have thrush without showing any symptoms, so thrush can be passed back and forth during sex. Thrush on the nipples can cause oral thrush for the baby during breastfeeding. Please contact your midwife or doctor for treatment if that is the case. Do not blow air into the vagina during oral sex; it can cause an air embolism, which is a serious medical condition.

Some factors that may reduce the frequency of sex toward the end of your pregnancy (from 37 weeks)

Your baby's head will descend further down into the pelvis, getting ready to be born. During your antenatal check, you may hear your midwife saying your baby's head is "engaged". Your baby's head being lower down in your pelvis, exerts more pressure, which may cause a pinching sensation in different parts of the pelvis, and pain deep in the vagina.

Sciatica is a sensation of pain, discomfort or numbness in your lower back, radiating through your buttock, leg or feet. It is caused by compression or inflammation of the sciatic nerve. Towards the end of your pregnancy, the womb causes pressure on the sciatic nerve as your baby grows bigger. If you suffer from sciatica, you need to talk to your midwife or GP for advice. The following can also help ease the pain:

- Physiotherapy;
- Bed rest;
- Applying a hot or cold compress;
- Change of position: try to lie on the side opposite the pain.

Symphysis pubis dysfunction (SPD) is separation of the pubic joint. You may experience pain in the pubic area, inner thigh and both buttocks. If you suffer from severe SPD, adapting to certain positions or movement during sex will be difficult due to pain.

What can you do?

- Speak to your midwife or GP for treatment and referral to a physiotherapist;
- Wear your support belt, usually provided by the physiotherapist;
- Avoid activities that will cause pain;
- Always have your knees together firmly when you turn over in bed or get out of bed;
- Have plenty of bed rest to take the body weight off the pelvis.

Not surprisingly, all the above discomforts towards the end of your pregnancy can impinge on your sexual desire and pleasure.

Hospital admissions

As a result of other pregnancy complications such as preeclampsia, pregnancy-induced hypertension, gestational diabetes or severe vomiting, you may be admitted to hospital for treatment. Your partner can visit you and send flowers and cards to show his affection (not all hospitals allow flowers, so please find out first). Once you are discharged home, you can continue your sex life as normal unless advised otherwise by your doctor.

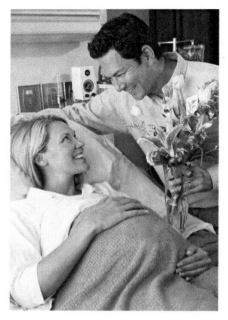

Husband giving flowers to wife on admission

Financial changes

Having a baby doesn't only bring about physical and psychological changes; there is also a financial demand. You may stop work or reduce your hours; your income will obviously drop as your expenditure increases; the maternity allowance may not be enough to cater for your growing and long-term needs. Your partner may need to work longer hours to bring in more money. Even couples without the added stress of a child find financial troubles to be a big killer of romance and intimacy.

You can do some things to help with financial concerns:

- Plan ahead and cut costs (could you do without the expensive jewellery or five-star holidays?);

- Buy only what you need, instead of everything you want;
- Don't buy too many baby clothes, as your baby will outgrow them very quickly. Instead try friends who have had babies, and look in charity shops for near-new clothing;
- Avoid buying too many or the most expensive baby accessories. Some, like a car seat, will be worth the expense, but you don't necessarily need a brand new stroller, for example;
- Keep an eye out for sales and bargains for any items;
- Charity shops are a good source for clothes, accessories and furniture. Some items may even be brand new;
- Always check second-hand items thoroughly before use.

Taking on more work during pregnancy

Housework, painting and decorating the baby's room and other activities can zap your energy. Moving into a new house can be tiring and stressful, too. There are, however, a few ways to reduce your workload:

- Space out the work; don't do it all in one day;
- Start early to avoid fitting everything in at the last minute;
- Ask for help from friends and family; they love you and will want to help out where they can;
- If you can afford it, employ someone to do the work.

Even doing one or two of the above suggestions, can reduce your stress levels and put you in the mood for love making.

There may be times when you will both experience intense, passionate lovemaking. Other times, you may experience calmness and be focused on your baby and the impending birth. These quiet moments will enable you, as a couple, to reconnect and continue to develop a relationship with your baby through ongoing preparation and discussion about how you are going to raise and support your baby when he or she is born.

CHAPTER 4

Positions you can adopt during pregnancy/Sex and romance in labour

As the pregnancy develops, your bump will get bigger and you will find it difficult to adopt certain positions during sex. For example, you will no longer be able to use the missionary position. Your stretching tummy may limit you from doing your usual acrobatics during sex. Many people at this stage end up abandoning sex altogether. Don't give up: explore new positions as an adventure to spice up your sex life. Give yourselves time to adjust to the new positions and adopt the ones you feel most comfortable in and which give you the greatest pleasure.

Lying on your side

You and your partner lie with him behind you. In this position, he will be able to hold you tight to his chest and kiss your neck. This position will also control thrusting and keep his weight off your tummy.

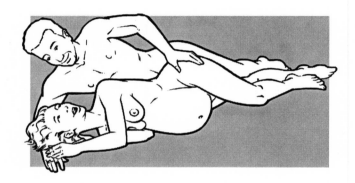

Woman on top

As your bump gets bigger, having your partner on top during intercourse can become uncomfortable for you. You being on top can be a satisfying position during late pregnancy. You can either face towards him or face away. He may also sit on a chair, or at the edge of the bed, whilst you sit on top, again either facing him or with your back to him. This position allows you to:

- Control the pace and be more comfortable;
- Control the depth of penetration while his hands are free to caress you;
- Support your weight on your knees or on the chair.

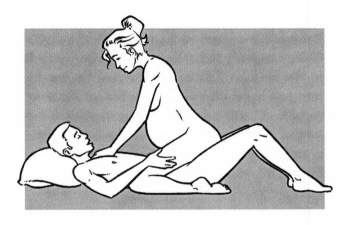

All fours position ("doggy")

Kneel down with your hands in front of you, so that your partner can penetrate your vagina from behind. He may penetrate more deeply in this position, so you must tell him if you are uncomfortable so that he can be gentle.

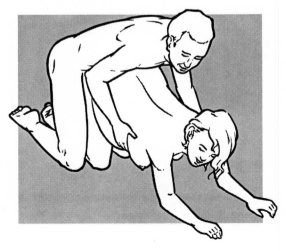

Spoon fashion

You should lie on your back (support your head with pillows to avoid lying completely flat) while your partner lies perpendicular to you, like the letter **T** facing you. Put your legs over his hips and open your legs to allow penetration. You can also lie on your side curled in a **C,** with your partner facing your back and curling around you. He then enters the vagina from behind while both of you are lying on your side. This intimate position is easy and comfortable. It is ideal when your bump becomes really large.

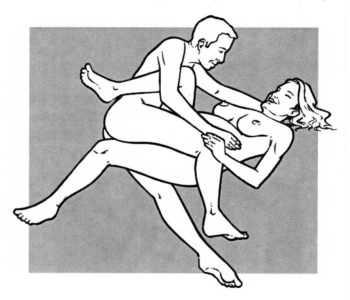

Making love on the stairs

This is best done close to the bottom of the stairs, so the risk of slipping is minimised. Kneel opposite the stairs. Your forearms should be well supported by one step. Your bump will fit nicely in the space between that step and the next step. Support your knee on the third step below. Your partner then inserts the penis in the vagina kneeling or standing behind you.

This position is good for all stages of pregnancy, particularly, during late pregnancy when your body is preparing to go into labour. The deep penetration of the penis will make it easier to deposit semen behind the cervix (the neck of the womb). The hormone-like substance in the semen called prostaglandins is believed to prepare and soften the cervix for labour.

Having sex to induce your labour at term; does it work?

Sexual intercourse at term as a mode of initiating labour is a popular belief. However, opinion is divided on the effectiveness of sex to induce labour at the end of pregnancy. There is not enough evidence to show whether sexual intercourse is effective or to show how it compares to other methods. More research is needed in this area. In my experience as a midwife, some women swear that it works, while others do not find it effective. Either way, midwives, doctors, friends and family may suggest sexual intercourse to bring on your labour when your baby is overdue; it is a non-medical method that allows you and your partner greater control over the process of attempting to start labour. Human sperm contains a high amount of prostaglandin, the hormone-like substance believed to soften the cervix and help labour to start. Nipple stimulation can also help to start your contractions. Oxytocin, the hormone that causes contractions (sometimes known as the love hormone) is released when breasts are stimulated.

> *Lilly, a first a time mum*
>
> *"I was comfortable with sex throughout the pregnancy. My labour started at 38 weeks, a few hours after having sex. I believe it works. It is worth making love; even if it does not start your labour, it helps. The activity is likely to make you feel happy, loved and relaxed."*

Nipple and clitoral stimulation in labour

Gentle rubbing or rolling of the nipple, or sucking to encourage contractions of the womb, is called nipple stimulation. The clitoris can also be stimulated along with the nipples. You are probably wondering how you can tolerate nipple or clitoral stimulation when you are in pain, stressed, and your partner feels helpless about the whole experience. It *is* possible, if you relax and prepare your mind for it.

Your contractions may stop or slow down during your labour. This may be due to stress or tiredness. Oxytocin is released in the body to bring on your contractions when your clitoris or nipples are stimulated. If your labour is uncomplicated, in the privacy of your home, you may try clitoral and nipple stimulation to induce some contractions. If you are having your baby in a birth centre, you may also be advised to try nipple stimulation before commencing artificial hormones.

I looked after Alice in a natural birth centre. Her contractions started disappearing during the second stage of labour. The couple had read about nipple and clitoral stimulation, so they asked if that truly works. I encouraged them to try it if they were comfortable doing so, and it worked for them. After several attempts, Alice started contracting again, and gave birth to a beautiful baby girl.

However, on other occasions, this method did not work for other women. Do not be disappointed if it does not work for you. It may be that your body is too exhausted from prolonged labour or your baby may be lying in an awkward position. Clitoral and nipple stimulation alone may not be enough to induce contractions; you may need the oxytocin drip for stronger and more frequent contractions.

Increased libido during labour

Most women get very distressed and restless in labour. Some may even push their partners away and not want to be touched, especially when they are getting closer to the birth and the contractions get stronger. However, a few women may have a strong desire to have sex while in labour with strong contractions.

Debra Pascali-Bonaro, a childbirth educator, created a film entitled "Orgasmic Birth", featuring real couples, being supported by midwives, obstetricians and other health professionals. She revealed that giving birth is a sexual and sensual experience. The hormone at play during labour, oxytocin, is the hormone released during sexual intercourse. It is normal to have some sexual sensation during labour. One of the women in the film said, "With good psychological preparation, the experience of contraction can be perceived as pleasure rather than pain. The body can translate the sensation as pleasure and experience orgasm during labour or childbirth."

During labour, especially the transition period (the end of first stage and the beginning of second stage), you may make sounds that are similar to the sounds during lovemaking and orgasm. There is an exquisite feeling of quaking and trembling in labour similar to that of lovemaking. In the video, some of the women said that they actually experienced orgasm during labour. Giving birth is part of a woman's sexual life; it is the continuation of what started in the bedroom to bring about the pregnancy.

The environment

Your spouse is used to your naked body only in the privacy of your home when you make love or have a bath together. As a couple you may find it embarrassing to be intimate in the presence of strangers in a hospital environment, with bright lights and strange noises. Staying at home is the best environment to be in during early labour, if there is no complication with the pregnancy. Most women with low-risk pregnancy still think the hospital is the safest place to be during labour "just in case" things go wrong. But staying in the hospital can in fact lead to unnecessary interference such as vaginal examinations, and electronic foetal monitoring, which can lead to a cascade of medical interventions.

It is fine to stay at home if:

- Your baby is moving;
- Your waters have not broken (ruptured membranes);
- You are not bleeding.

The midwives are at the end of the phone to give advice if you have any concerns. Stay at home as long as possible until you have strong regular contractions (coming every three minutes and lasting for a minute, especially if it is your first baby).

In the privacy of your home, you have the opportunity to express your love, touch and kiss and be intimate without any interference. You can dim the lights, play music or do anything that can help you to relax. When your mind and body are relaxed, your labour progresses well. Couples who live with other family members or have other siblings may not achieve this easily at home. When you go into active labour you may wish to use a birthing centre, which is like home from home. Do not be despondent, though, if you have complications and cannot be at home or access a birthing centre. The midwives can still try to minimise any disturbances in the delivery ward, and create a calm and sensitive environment for your labour.

Choosing your partner as your birthing coach

In the United Kingdom, men are expected to be in the delivery room when their partner is giving birth. In other cultures, it is the opposite: the woman's mother, aunt or other female relative is the one who provides support. While some women may prefer their mother or friend to be with them, others may insist their partner be present.

Some midwives have observed that some women are able to delay giving birth until their partner arrives. This may well be a coincidence, or it may be that his presence allows her to relax and finally give birth, possibly because of the love they share between them. Some men are excited and look forward to being present at the birth. You may feel safe, secure and relaxed when your partner is present. You may find it helpful to hold his hands and hug him.

He is there to support you and help you have the best possible experience. A good birth partner is someone who:

- Wants to be there and is not forced to be there;
- Can look after himself and not need attention;
- Knows what you want;
- Will empathise with you;
- Accepts that you may change your mind and that he will need to go with the flow;
- Asks questions, expresses concerns and works together with the midwives and doctors.

I have observed that most men are calm and supportive, even if they are nervous. Others cope by withdrawing into themselves and occupy themselves with reading (they may not make any sense of what they are reading, mind you!). The majority of men feel helpless and frustrated that their partner is in pain and there is nothing or very little they can do. Others are not sure what they are expected to do. A few of them are squeamish and will prefer not to be present. In this case, you can bring a trusted friend, a doula (a birth companion who provides support to the mother before, during and after birth), or a family member to support both of you.

Some women feel, if they tell their partner to stay out of the room, he may be offended; but it is all right to ask your partner to wait outside while you are being examined or giving birth to your baby if you do not feel comfortable. It may be that you do not want your partner to see "down there" when you are giving birth, or he may feel awkward or embarrassed when the midwife is performing a vaginal examination. To avoid this, he can stand at the top end of the bed, hold your hand, give you eye contact and whisper encouraging words in your ears while you are giving birth.

Every couple will feel differently about the entire process of labour; do what makes you feel comfortable. Both of you need to discuss these issues well in advance and prepare yourselves psychologically before your labour starts. If this is discussed when neither of you are stressed, then whatever the decision is, you will both be comfortable with it.

If you and your partner have a misunderstanding or your relationship is strained, you may not want him present at the birth. His presence in the labour room can cause emotional distress if the problem is not resolved. It is important to try and resolve any emotional conflicts if possible, before your labour starts. Letting go of the anger and pain will help you to labour better, because you will be able to relax and be present in the moment.

Your partner expressing love and giving you support in labour

As with any life-changing event, the extent to which you feel supported, listened to and involved during your labour will affect your feelings about your birth experience. Continuous support will enable you to cope better with your labour. Research by the Midwives' Information and Resource Service (MIDDIRS) shows that effective support can:

1. Reduce your chance of using pain-relieving drugs.
2. Result in fewer Caesarean sections, or forceps or ventouse (vacuum-assisted) births.

3. Reduce dissatisfaction with the childbirth experience.

Here are some of the things your partner can do to support you:

*   Simply saying encouraging words can help;
*   Massaging your lower back, if appropriate. It may not be possible to massage in some complicated cases. Massage usually helps to ease the lower back pain, especially when the baby is in a back-to-back position;

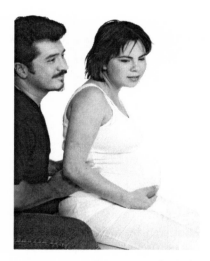

*A man massaging his partner's lower back
in early labour to ease discomfort*

*   Playing music of your choice;
*   Kissing, hugs and gentle strokes;
*   Advocate for you by asking the midwife and doctors if something is unclear;

- Wipe your sweat and encourage you to eat and drink if your labour is normal.

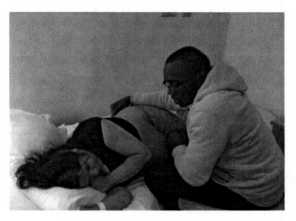

A man massaging his wife in advanced labour

Tips for partners

Your partner may find it helpful if you talk to her by saying loving and encouraging words like: well done, you are doing a good job, I love you. On the other hand, she may find it annoying or disruptive, especially during contractions. She may withdraw into herself during labour and prefer the room to be quiet and undisturbed. At the peak of a contraction, she may not wish to be touched. She may find it irritating and uncomfortable. She may even scream and tell you to shut up. She may swear or use colourful language even if swearing has never been part of her vocabulary. Do not take it personally; show understanding and support her any way she wants you to. She does not mean to be rude or ungrateful; most women are usually apologetic after the event.

Does observing the birth of the baby put men off sex?

Most women are concerned that if their partner watches the birth of their baby, the memory of the stretching vagina by the baby's head may affect them psychologically during lovemaking. The vagina is an amazing organ! It has the ability to deliver the baby and go back to normal after the baby is born. It works like elastic – it can stretch and retract. Routine pelvic floor exercises will help to make the vaginal muscles stronger and firmer after your baby is born. You can start your pelvic floor exercise within 24 hours after the birth.

The majority of women also get very worried and embarrassed about opening their bowels when the baby is being born. Some find it undignified in front of their partner. Other women may be worried that all these things will, again, put their partner off making love with them later on.

To prevent this from happening, some women go to the extent of not eating when they are about to go into labour. This will only make you feel weak and have no energy to cope with your labour. Usually, when you are about to go into labour, you will naturally open your bowels a few days before your labour starts. This may not always happen, though, especially if you are constipated. Drink plenty of fluids, eat enough fibre and enjoy fruits and vegetables. Gentle exercise can often help you empty your bowels before you go into labour.

When the delivery of your baby is getting closer, you may feel a strong sensation to open your bowels. This is usually your baby's head pressing against your back passage (rectum), giving you the urge to push. This sensation is very strong when your baby is in the back-to-back (occipito-posterior) position. It is natural and beyond your control if you end up having a bowel movement. It may feel odd, but there really is no need to be embarrassed or worried about it.

Did you know?

Opening your bowels during the second stage of labour is a good sign. It means your baby is close to being born. The midwives and doctors will deal with it sensitively and professionally.

It is a widespread belief among women that during sex, the man may have flashbacks of the gaping birth canal and the whole labour experience. He may have it ingrained in his mind that the vagina is bigger and will not go back to normal. The truth is that all men vary in their sexual desire following pregnancy and birth.

After talking to a lot of men, I discovered that most of them were more concerned with the wellbeing of the mother and baby. After going through the pregnancy with you and reading the books, they have a good understanding of the female body and they know that the vagina eventually returns to its normal state after birth. Most men are rather grateful for what their wife has to go through to give birth to their baby. It makes them appreciate and love her even more.

Some of the men admitted that observing the process of birth had a negative impact on their sex drive. As it is common knowledge that men are usually moved by what they see (and women by what they feel), it follows that the sight of their partner giving birth may put some off sex. The following factors might also quench your partner's desire for sex temporarily:

- *Observing the midwife / doctor perform the cut at the perineum (episiotomy), to aid the delivery of the baby;*
- *The doctor inserting the suction cup or forceps to deliver the baby (instrumental delivery);*
- *Vaginal examinations;*
- *Stitching the tears / episiotomy;*
- *Bleeding;*
- *Seeing his loved one distressed and screaming in pain;*
- *Worried that they may reinjure your episiotomy wound.*

Darren's experience

"The experience I had in the delivery room, coupled with what I had read and heard, affected my desire for sex initially. It took us about six months before we made love. I felt Vera needed more time to heal. We were occupied with getting used to the new baby, sleepless nights and exhaustion. It felt strange, the first night we made love. I felt the vagina was 'loose'; I guess it was my imagination rather than the reality. As the baby grew and settled, life began to feel normal again. We now enjoy sex as we did before our daughter Sasha came along."

What Nicolas had to say:

Nicolas, a father of two, said, "Watching the birth did not put me off having sex with my wife. Instead, I appreciated and respected her more for what she had to go through to give birth to our precious baby. We carried on with our sex life as normal when she recovered."

Interesting facts about sex and labour

During labour, women make spontaneous sounds e.g. groaning and screaming, as the labour gets intense.	*During sexual intercourse, women make spontaneous sounds like scream or make noise to express pleasure during their climax or orgasm.*
During labour, the vagina lubricates and opens, preparing for the baby to pass through.	*During sexual intercourse the vagina lubricates, ready for the penis to penetrate.*
The love hormone oxytocin is released during labour, to bring on contractions.	*The love hormone oxytocin is also released during orgasm.*
During labour, the womb contracts rhythmically (the contractions in labour are far more intense and cause the neck of the womb to open (cervical dilatation)).	*During sex, the womb contracts rhythmically, but it is painless.*
There is a feeling of intense emotion, vulnerability and sensitivity during labour.	*During lovemaking, most women feel emotional, vulnerable and sensitive.*
Childbirth involves intimacy and bonding with your partner.	*Lovemaking involves intimacy and bonding with your partner.*
During labour, your body is exposed to the person assisting the birth.	*During sex, your body is exposed to your partner.*

Labour can be disrupted when the environment is not conducive, such as poor temperature, noise, bright lights, intrusion.	*Sex can be disrupted by noise – for example, the new baby crying – and intrusion.*
Social inhibitions go out of the window towards the end of labour as the contractions gets stronger. For example, a woman who is shy or who feels uneasy removing her clothes for a vaginal examination will no longer care.	*Social inhibitions cease to be a barrier when a woman is about to reach climax during sex. A woman may be shy during foreplay, especially with a new partner. As her emotions take over, and she begins to enjoy, she does not show any shyness as she reaches her climax.*
Labour does not progress well if there are undesirable feelings such as fear, anger, stress, anxiety.	*The enjoyment of lovemaking can be dampened by fear, anger, stress, anxiety, etc.*
Labour progresses well and it is satisfying when you surrender your mind and body to it.	*Sex is most pleasurable when you relax and surrender your body and mind to it.*

CHAPTER 5

Attitudes, behaviours, myths, cultural practices and beliefs about sex and childbirth

Culture, religion and strict moral codes have a significant influence on people's attitudes in relation to sex during pregnancy and after the birth. In some instances, advice from family and friends, based on cultural practices, may hold more weight than advice from health professionals. Some ethnic minority groups are afraid to lose their cultural practices and beliefs, so they ensure that these are instilled in their children who are born and raised outside their home countries.

There are certain cultural practices that are fading away as people become more westernised and receive information from healthcare providers. As people integrate into a different society, they may lose touch with their traditional practices. In the UK, the introduction of antenatal classes brought a surge of new information to mums and dads-to-be. The subject of sex during pregnancy, which was not mentioned in the past, is now formally included in parents' education programmes, even though it may not be emphasised as much as other topics like pain relief or breastfeeding.

In today's multicultural society, where marriages between cultures are common, it is important to create public awareness by highlighting some of the cultural beliefs surrounding sex and childbirth. The examples of cultural and religious practices given here are by no means exhaustive; the information given is based on feedback from women and their partners, members of the public, friends, family, professional colleagues and several secondary sources.

Cultural beliefs

China

During the initial stages (usually the first trimester) of pregnancy, women are not allowed to lift, do any heavy-duty work or have any sexual relations with their husband, to avoid miscarriage. The first month after delivery is called *Zuo Yuezi*, meaning "doing the month". During this period, the woman's behaviour in relation to diet, sexual activity and hygiene is determined by tradition. The common view is that sexual activity should be forbidden after the birth (postpartum period), for several reasons:

1. The woman is weak, she has no energy.
2. She is concentrating on looking after the baby, and needs rest.
3. The wound has not yet healed.
4. She is still bleeding, and intercourse can cause infection.

This period ranges from one to three months, and the healthcare professionals and traditional medicine practitioners support the practice.

Africa

In certain parts of Africa, when a baby is born covered in "white stuff" (vernix caseosa), it is believed that the couple had sex shortly before labour and released the semen over the baby's skin. Others believe that vernix is dirty and makes the baby smell if it is not washed off. As a result, the new baby is washed until all the vernix is removed.

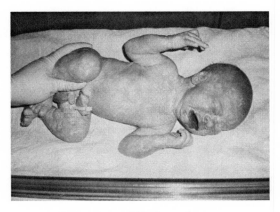

Five-minute-old baby with vernix

Did you know?

Vernix caseosa is a natural moisturiser that protects the baby's skin. When a baby receives his first bath, there is no need to vigorously wash the "white stuff" off. It will naturally rub off with time.

89

In certain parts of Nigeria, it is believed that if a woman has intercourse while still breastfeeding, the semen will travel to the breast milk and may cause the baby to suffer from certain illnesses.

Did you know?

Sexual intercourse while breastfeeding does not cause diseases. The semen does not travel to the breast milk, so it is safe to enjoy sex whilst you are still breastfeeding.

Traditionally, in some African countries such as Ghana, once a woman gives birth, she moves to her maternal home for some weeks to be supported by her wider family. She is excused from household chores and is supported with the baby's care. She is well fed to regain her strength, and also for successful breastfeeding. The man visits his wife, the new baby and the in-laws, but returns to the marital home to sleep.

As much as this practice is to support the new mum to rest and care for the baby, the hidden agenda is to prevent her from having sex too soon with her husband. The idea is to give her body time to heal, especially if she had any perineal tears. It is also a way of promoting family planning, by preventing her from falling pregnant again too soon. This practice is rapidly changing due to migration, transcultural influences, mixed marriages, and the institution of the nuclear family. The mother or mother-in-law may be invited instead to the couple's own home after the baby is born.

The first sexual encounter after the birth is usually associated with pain. It is not uncommon, especially among the Akans in Ghana, for friends and acquaintances to teasingly ask new mums and dads, "W'ate wo meko"? ("Have you plucked your chilli peppers?"), a metaphor meaning have you had your first sexual intercourse since the birth?

In Ghana, and in some other cultures around the world, the new mum may douche, insert substances like finely ground herbs and ginger in the vagina to keep it "dry". This intervention is believed to aid quick healing and to restore the "tightness" of the vagina for sex. Some women believe these agents strengthen the body, prevent thrush, and tone the pelvic floor muscles. They also believe it can prevent or treat sexually transmitted infections, vaginal infections, itching and discharge.

However, it is generally accepted in the UK that douching and using herbs or other agents to cleanse or dry the vagina may be harmful. Through health education campaigns, women in Africa and other countries are becoming increasingly aware that these practices are unsafe.

A healthy vagina contains some bacteria and other organisms called vaginal flora. The normal acidity of the vagina keeps the amount of bacteria down. Douching can upset this delicate balance. Nor do the substances used cure or prevent diseases. Research shows that women who douche regularly have more vaginal health problems than those who do not. Douching can also cause irritation and spread existing vaginal infection up into the uterus, fallopian tubes and ovaries. A dry vagina may cause more friction and pain during sexual intercourse.

In some parts of the world, sex is deemed to be for child-bearing purposes only. Certain groups believe that having sex during pregnancy drains energy from the mother. Sex is discouraged on the grounds that the mother's energy should go to her baby and not used for pleasure. Contrary to this view, other cultures believe that to produce a strong and healthy baby, the expectant couple should have sex frequently. It is believed that the foetus comes from the mother's blood (as indicated by the cessation of menstruation during pregnancy) and the father's bone (referring to the semen). Therefore, to produce a strong and healthy baby the couple should have sex frequently.

Some African cultures believe that the baby will swallow the semen if the parents engage in sex during pregnancy. If the baby sneezes after birth, it is associated with the fact that the baby had swallowed a lot of semen. This, of course, has no scientific basis.

Religious beliefs

Muslims believe that a woman should not have sex when she is still bleeding. The couple must abstain from sex during the postnatal period until 40 days after the birth, when the bleeding is expected to have stopped. A woman is required to have a ritual bath following sexual intercourse, before she can pray. Muslims also avoid sex during Ramadan.

If the couple are Orthodox Jews, a husband and wife are not permitted to have sex if she is bleeding from her uterus, and while this usually means during her menstrual period, it also applies after the birth. However, when a woman is pregnant, it is permissible for them to have sex anytime – and in Judaism, sex is the woman's right, not the man's, so it is his duty to please his wife.

Christianity has no definitive rules about sex during fasting. To have sex or not is to be determined by agreement between the couple. Some Christians avoid sex during their fasting period because they believe that they need to focus on their prayers and do not want any distractions. Some believe abstaining from sex means they are pure and holy in the presence of God; others may have no energy for lovemaking because they may feel too weak or hungry during a long fast.

Some Seventh-day Adventist couples avoid having sex after sunset on Friday nights, because they observe the Sabbath on Saturday and regard it as a day of rest. They believe having sex is a form of using energy: it can make you sweat, and therefore it is regarded as work.

Within the Roman Catholic religion, contraception is a central issue. The Catholic Church strongly disallows artificial birth control methods such as condoms, pills, injections and sterilisation. Couples who wish to have children are only expected to have sex during the infertile period of the woman's menstrual cycle. Other natural family-planning methods that the Catholic Church generally approves of include the rhythm method, the standard day method, and basal body temperature charting. This rule also applies to couples who have just had a new baby and don't want to fall pregnant too soon.

Attitudes and behaviours towards sex

People feel and behave differently towards sex depending on their cultural and religious background or how they have been socialised. Some women find it embarrassing to talk to their partner about sex or approach him for sex, or introduce any new sexual practice. She feels she may be regarded as promiscuous. In most relationships, people form a habit whereby one person initiates most or all of the sex. It may be that one partner is shy, not interested, embarrassed, or does not enjoy sex. Some women may also feel it is the man's duty to initiate sex all the time.

Your partner initiating sex can make you feel beautiful, attractive and desired, as some women have testified. However,

93

it should not be one-sided – you should also initiate sex if you want. Some men wish their partners would initiate sex sometimes because they also want to feel attractive and desired. If he is always the one approaching you, he may feel he is risking rejection in case you are not in the mood. He may even think you are not interested in him, so he will subconsciously (or consciously) put his urges aside. You may then think he isn't interested, and suffer in silence.

During your pregnancy, the partner you know to be manic when it comes to sex may suddenly change and withdraw. As your bump grows bigger, the pregnancy will become more real to him. Among other reasons, he may be afraid to hurt the baby, as we have discussed previously. He may start making excuses to avoid sex. His lack of interest can make you feel frustrated and rejected.

It takes constant open communication to understand what your spouse desires. Presume your partner does not know how to satisfy you, and vice versa, and that you need to ask each other. It is important to discuss sex because men and women have fundamentally different sexual needs, and, especially during pregnancy, these needs may change. Ongoing heart-to-heart talks will help both of you to meet your sexual needs.

> *Reena, a 29-year-old mother of two, said, "I feel embarrassed to approach my husband for sex. I do enjoy sex and I feel good when Philip approaches me for sex, but I simply could not bring myself to initiate it. It has always been like that, from the beginning of our relationship. I know Philip was not happy about it because he complained a few times. We had sex only a few times during the pregnancy. Even when I desired sex, I could not ask for it. Reading romantic books has given me more insight about lovemaking. I can now approach him for sex when I feel like it.*

Infidelity

Some women may turn inward about midway through their pregnancy, and her partner may feel that he is no longer important. Some men react by seeking another woman and initiating an affair. Some women may equally feel rejected when the man constantly turns her down for sex. On rare occasions a pregnant woman may look elsewhere to meet her sexual needs because she may feel frustrated and think her partner no longer desires he r. Some women may be worried that if they do not satisfy their partner at home, he will go out and cheat. Even if they are not ready or unwell, they may force themselves, just to please him and keep him at home. This should not be necessary if you and your partner have honest conversations about your ideas for sex and your expectations in terms of fidelity.

Kofi and Agnes have been together for three years. Kofi said, "Agnes lost interest in sex when she became pregnant. She became very moody and irritable. We could never finish a conversation without arguing. She couldn't even bear the sight of me. I felt rejected, frustrated and unloved. I found myself having an affair with my ex- girlfriend. After a while, I felt guilty and stopped."

If you love each other and care for your unborn baby, you will rise above any challenges you may face and talk to each other about your sexual and emotional needs and how you feel. You may also seek sexual counselling together. Infidelity will only compound problems in the relationship, and in some cases you may end up apart, even before the baby arrives. In practical terms, if you contract a sexually transmitted infection, you can infect your partner and even your unborn baby.

> *Did you know?*
>
> *Sexually transmitted infections can affect your baby. Syphilis can cross the placenta and infect the baby before it is born. Chlamydia, gonorrhoea and genital herpes can be transmitted during the birth. HIV can be transmitted in the womb, during the birth and during breastfeeding. The doctor or midwife can offer you blood test counselling and treatment. Alternatively, you can attend a sexual health clinic for blood tests and advice.*

Breastfeeding

Some people do not like seeing women breastfeed in public. They find it embarrassing, a form of exhibitionism, or even disgusting behaviour. Some women decline breastfeeding because they see their breasts as a sexual organ rather than as a food-source for the baby. They feel breastfeeding the baby will make the breasts saggy and unattractive. But breast changes occur as soon as you become pregnant; avoiding breastfeeding may not make any difference. Some women feel good about breastfeeding – apart from bonding with your baby and other numerous health benefits for the baby, some women wish to have bigger breasts. The increase in breast size during pregnancy and breastfeeding makes them feel sexier.

Chapter 6

Resuming sex after the birth of your baby

Resuming sex depends on individual circumstances and when you feel ready. It is very common for your sex drive to decrease after childbirth. Your first priority has shifted from your partner to your baby. Your body is adapting to the physical and psychological changes, the lack of sleep, and the massive adjustment that a new baby demands. You may be too sore or exhausted to think about sex. Both you and your partner may be apprehensive and anxious about resuming sex. You are not alone – most couples feel the same way. You may be wondering if sex will feel the same as before. You may be worried that it will be painful rather than pleasurable. Some women cannot bear the idea of resuming sex after childbirth and may resist their partner until it reaches crises point. In my interviews, some couples disclosed that it took them a year to resume sex. Other couples said they eased back into sexual intercourse without any problems – even before the six-week postnatal check-up with their GP.

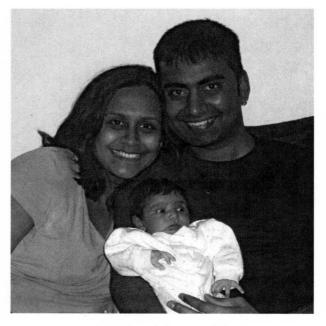

A couple and their new baby

When can you start?

Whether you give birth vaginally or by Caesarean section, your body needs time to heal. Your midwife or obstetrician may recommend that you wait six weeks before resuming sex. The idea is to allow enough time for your cervix to close and any tears or repaired episiotomy wounds to heal. The postnatal bleeding (lochia) would also have stopped by then. If the wound does not heal properly before sex, the perineum can break down and become infected. Women who do not sustain perineal tears are more likely to resume sex earlier because there is no fear of pain.

Perineal and vaginal tears

(For more information, see Chapter 2, pages 45-46): Classification of tears).

Women who have perineal tears and stitches after the birth may feel anxious about resuming sex due to the fear of pain. Initially, your vulva and perineum may be swollen and bruised. It will feel different from how you normally feel for a few days. You are not alone. Some women believe the birth canal becomes abnormal after the birth.

Lindsey said, "I felt as though my vagina was not normal, and therefore I went off sex for a while. Thanks to my partner, Bob, because he cherishes and loves me – his constant support and positive comments helped me to feel good and open up for sex again."

Katherine and Glenn

Katherine and Glenn had their beautiful baby girl at 6:30 a.m. on a Saturday morning. After stitching Katherine's perineal tear, I started talking about perineal care and when they could resume sex. There was a broad smile on Glenn's face, like the sun rising at dawn. Out of curiosity, I asked why he was smiling. He said, "After a long wait throughout the pregnancy, I now have the green light to start having sex again when Katherine recovers." Katherine replied, "After what I've just gone through, pushing the baby out, the last thing on my mind is sex. In fact I don't think I will fall pregnant again." Katherine was also worried that the stitches would make sex very painful. I advised them to make compromises and to consider other innovative forms of lovemaking.

Some women have reported that their perineal pain lasted six months or more. If you end up with an episiotomy or tears, you should:

- Tell the midwife or doctor how you feel. If the stitches are sore and uncomfortable they may offer you some pain relief to sooth it;
- Do your pelvic floor exercises regularly;
- Keep the area dry after washing with plain water, and change your pad regularly to avoid infection. Tea tree oil (4-6 drops dissolved in milk and added to your bath water) has been found to be soothing and to aid healing. (Check first to ensure you are not sensitive to this essential oil by testing it on the inside of your elbow or behind your ear);
- Try to avoid constipation to prevent any strain on your stitches and minimise discomfort. You may find it daunting to open your bowels for fear that your stitches may rip apart. As a result, you may stop yourself from going to the toilet for several days. This will cause constipation and make the situation worse. Drink plenty of fluids and eat fruit and vegetables to help free your bowels. If this does not work, speak to your GP about other options;
- Wait for the wound to heal before resuming sex. If you touch the area and it does not hurt, sex may not hurt.

Unfortunately, there have been instances where women have been forced or pressured by their partner to have sex too soon, causing the stitches to rip apart or the wound to be infected. You should *never* feel under pressure or forced to have sex – it is an abuse of your body and soul. If you feel under any psychological or physical threat from your partner, don't suffer in silence. Talk to your midwife, GP or a domestic abuse counsellor. Dr De Angelis says that if you allow a man to treat you disrespectfully it creates a negative self-esteem cycle.

The negative self-esteem cycle

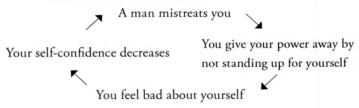

Body image after childbirth

1. Weak vaginal muscle tone

Laxity of the birth canal can occur as a result of having several children, delivering large babies, or having difficult deliveries. The vaginal walls become lax and may not return to their pre-pregnancy state. You may feel embarrassed during intercourse due to too little muscle tone. In most cases, routine pelvic floor exercise helps to resolve this. However, if the problem is severe, pelvic floor exercises alone may not be enough. A specialised surgical tightening and rejuvenation of the vagina, perineum and the supporting muscles may be beneficial. This is done by removing excess vaginal lining and tightening the surrounding soft tissues and muscles. There are skilled surgeons who are specialists in performing the procedure with good results. (Note:

this procedure is not for every woman, so be aware of the risks and ensure that your surgeon is qualified in this type of operation).

2. Vaginal tags and perineal breakdown

Unfortunately, in a minority of women the skin of the perineum may break down. Others may have extra skin hanging, perineal pain, vulva and vaginal stenosis (loss of flexibility), and sexual dysfunction in the months following vaginal delivery. If you experience any of these problems, do not suffer in silence. Seek medical advice immediately. Your GP should refer you to hospital for secondary repair. The good news is that most secondary repairs have a good success rate.

3. Fistula caused by childbirth injuries

A fistula is when a hole develops between the vagina and the bladder and/or the rectum, resulting in steady leakage of urine and faeces. It is a childbirth injury that can have a massive impact on the new mother. Fistula is very rare in Western countries.

Obstetric fistula is believed to be most common among young women experiencing their first pregnancy, especially in regions where early marriage is the norm. It is caused by several days of obstructed labour without timely medical intervention, such as Caesarean section, to relieve the pressure.

Because of the lack of understanding and social stigma, women with a fistula frequently suffer in silence. Early repair and treatment is critical. It prevents a cycle of stigma and discrimination that often leads to dependency, disempowerment and a loss of self-esteem for women.

4. Weight gain

Celebrity culture and the media have a great influence on the general public's sense of how we should look. As women, we are constantly bombarded with images of the "perfect body": the tall, size zero models. Most women influenced by celebrity fashion trends, after having their baby, embark on crash exercise programmes and quick dieting regimens to get back to the so-called "perfect" body shape.

As I said before, weight gain and body-shape change is normal during pregnancy. It takes time to return to your normal shape after the birth. If you want to return to your pre-pregnancy weight and shape quickly, your self-esteem and confidence may be affected if this does not happen as desired. When you get naked around your partner, you may be self-conscious, scared that if he looks at you he will discover your stretch marks, darkened skin and flabby tummy. You may not feel sexually attractive and may lose interest in sex. At this time, with a new baby to care for, it is better to eat healthily and exercise safely so as to lose weight steadily. Learn to love your body as an expression of feminine beauty. Your body has changed for a good reason and you've brought a new life to the world. Embrace that.

Tips for partners
- *Support your partner to lose weight in a healthy way and when she is ready;*
- *Avoid making negative comments like mentioning her "wobbly tummy" or "chubby thighs". You may be joking or trying to be endearing, but remember: words are powerful. These comments will not make her feel confident about herself;*

> • *Let her know that she is still desired at a time when she may be feeling less than desirable;*
> • *Avoid putting pressure on her to get back to her original weight prior to pregnancy and childbirth.*

Generally, after several months you will lose the excess weight. Here are some tips for getting back to your pre-pregnancy shape:

1. Eating healthy food along with exercise can help to speed the process.
2. Having a walk together while "daddy" carries the baby can be romantic and burn calories at the same time.
3. Push the baby in the pram for school runs and short distances instead of driving.
4. While daddy watches the baby, you can go to the local park for cycling – and get some alone time.
5. Some gyms have free child-care if you can afford to join.
6. Avoid shopping at the supermarket while hungry, and stick to a planned list of groceries from menus for the week.

Bleeding (lochia)

After the baby is born, it is normal to have a heavy period for the first few days. The amount reduces after three to four days and the colour changes to brown and eventually to a normal white discharge. The time the bleeding stops varies between women. Some women may bleed lightly for up to a month. Some women may also spot for several weeks. It is generally medically recommended that the bleeding stops before you start sexual intercourse, in order to prevent infection.

Fear of falling pregnant again too soon

You may be worried about getting pregnant again too soon. This can make you feel tense during lovemaking, or you may decide to abstain altogether. This feeling is normal, and it *is* possible to fall pregnant before your first period after the birth of your baby.

When your period re-starts varies considerably among women, and can depend on how you feed your baby. If you are not breastfeeding, your first period (menstruation) can start as early as five to eight weeks after the birth. Breastfeeding mums may not have another period until they have stopped. You can get pregnant again as early as 21 days after your baby is born. You can become pregnant even if you are breastfeeding. Breastfeeding is only effective when you haven't had any periods and are breastfeeding when the baby is less than 6 months old. The baby should breastfeed every two to four hours, with no missed feeds. To stick to this routine, you should not give your baby any food or drink apart from breast milk.

Make sure you decide on a reliable family planning method before resuming sex. Effective contraception will put your mind at rest during sex, because a lot of unplanned pregnancies happen in the first few months after the birth. The majority of women release an egg (ovulation) about two weeks before their period. You should get contraception advice from your GP, midwife or family planning clinic. The family planning nurse will assess you and help you choose what will be suitable for you and your partner. While you wait to sort out your birth control, you may need to have a back-up plan (such as condoms). Condoms can be obtained in any supermarket, chemist, general health centre or family planning clinic. Some couples find that putting on a condom is very sensual and reminds them of their early sexual experiences together.

Exhaustion

The first few weeks of looking after a new baby are exhausting, especially when you have not recovered from giving birth. Apart from the routine housework, you will need to feed, change the baby and attend to his or her general needs. Exhaustion from these activities will suppress your desire for sex. Get your partner involved in bathing the baby and changing the baby's nappies. Share the workload so that you can both conserve some energy for lovemaking.

List of numerous activities to be fitted into 24 hours

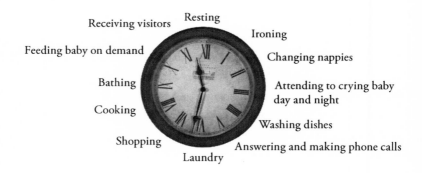

Receiving visitors

Resting

Ironing

Feeding baby on demand

Changing nappies

Bathing

Attending to crying baby day and night

Cooking

Washing dishes

Shopping

Answering and making phone calls

Laundry

Traumatic birth experience

Most women overcome their pain, fear and anxiety of labour and birth when they see their bundle of joy and realise that all is well. For others, the traumatic events surrounding the birth experience remain in their mind. This may affect their relationship with their partner and baby. If you experience this, you should consider the following suggestions:

- Do not ignore how you are feeling;
- Open up by talking to your partner. Be honest, so that he can support you;
- Inform your doctor or midwife of your need for support. You may need counselling to overcome the emotional distress.

Baby blues / postnatal depression

On the third or fourth day after having your baby, you may get tearful, feel "flat", or be unsure of yourself. This is because you may be battling sleeplessness or tiredness while responding to the demanding needs of your newborn. All of these issues can make you lose interest in sex, not to mention lose interest in yourself and your baby. Most women feel the same, so you are not alone. You will feel better with tender loving care, rest and support from your partner and other family members.

As many as eight out of ten women get the "baby blues"; however, some women (about ten per cent of new mothers) get postnatal depression, which usually encompasses much stronger feelings of helplessness, hopelessness and incompetence to correctly care for their baby. These issues are real and may last for several months; therefore, you should speak to your GP if you feel this way. You may not notice this, but a partner or family member may, so listen to them – they are only trying to help. Many women with postnatal depression may need antidepressants to help them overcome this period in their lives.

Tips for partners

If your partner is in an unfavourable mood, it can be tempting to follow suit. You know your partner best – when you notice any changes in mood, do not ignore them. Asking how your partner feels will show that you care. Taking up as much of the burden as you can will show that you're a capable partner.

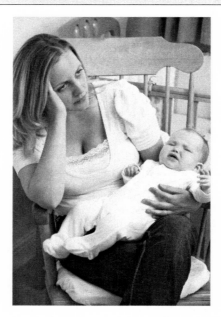

A mum not showing any interest in her crying baby

What can be done?

1. Do not try to be a "superwoman". Try to do less and make sure you don't get over-tired; get your partner involved in the care of your newborn.

2. Talk to your midwife, health visitor or GP about how you feel so that they can give you professional help.

3. Make friends with other women or couples who are expecting or have just had a baby.

4. Regular exercise can boost your mood and help you to feel less isolated. You may find it easier to do this with other people, such as other new mums or at the gym.

5. Find someone you can talk to. If you do not have a close friend, you can contact organisations that can help (see Resources section).

Lack of privacy

After a birth, some women may leave their home for a few weeks to go and stay with their parents. If that is not possible, a family member, usually the mother, will come to the couple's house to support them. In certain cultures, the presence of another person can restrict romantic and sexual activities. You may feel embarrassed to show affection in the presence of your in-laws. It may be perceived as disrespectful. You may even worry that you will be overheard. Having someone around is like a double-edged sword: getting a helping hand can be advantageous; however, if the person becomes controlling and interfering rather than supportive, it can cause stress and frustration – two things which are not good for rekindling romance.

Sharing the room with the baby and other siblings

You may feel that the newborn can hear and understand you when you make love, or that the baby may wake up while you are at the peak of having fun. But this will not be because the baby is aware of what is happening: it may be feeding time, the nappy may need changing, or maybe the baby wants to be cuddled. If there is an older child, you may be worried that he might wake up and walk into your bedroom while you are making love. With these thoughts niggling at the back of your mind, it will be difficult to relax. You may feel you need to reduce your screaming, groaning or talking, and you may opt for a "quickie" as a result.

A newborn baby will be oblivious to an activity such as lovemaking. Make sure the baby is well fed and has a dry nappy, before settling down to sleep. Keep the door shut if you are concerned that an older child might barge in. Start training the child at an early age to knock on Mummy and Daddy's door and to wait for a response before coming in.

Breastfeeding

As new parents, you will be bombarded with the advantages of breastfeeding before the arrival of the baby. Some of the benefits include: better bonding with the baby; that it protects the baby against infections; that your milk has the perfect blend of nutrients; and there are many more reasons besides. As parents, you want the best for your baby, and even the World Health Organization recommends that mums should breastfeed exclusively for the first six months, and then continue for two years.

Most husbands are supportive of breastfeeding for the above reasons. However, your partner may perceive you as a nursing mother rather than a lover. Dr Armin Brott, a father of two daughters and the author of *Expectant Father*, revealed that sometimes dads may experience:

- A slight feeling of resentment towards the baby who has come between him and his partner;
- A fear that it's going to get harder to bond and develop a relationship with his child;
- A sense of inadequacy that nothing he could do will compete with the breast;
- A sense of relief when the baby is weaned, because he will finally have a chance to get back in touch with his partner physically, to put her nipples and breasts back into the lovemaking mix.

As a lactating mum, you may feel your body is divided into two sections: the lower part is for your partner, for sex, while the top half is for the baby to breastfeed. For some women, the breasts play a major role during lovemaking. Not being able to use them to the maximum due to pain, engorgement, or nipple cracks, makes the whole idea of having sex undesirable. Apart from the reasons mentioned, the following factors may also reduce your desire for sex.

- You may feel guilty and in conflict about having sexual feelings for your partner while breastfeeding your baby;

- High prolactin levels (the hormone responsible for releasing breast milk) and low oestrogen levels may affect your libido;
- Tiredness caused by feeding day and night may impact on your sex drive;
- Your need for intimacy is being met by the baby.

The "love hormone" (oxytocin) releases milk from the breast during orgasm. Milk ejection during intercourse may cause embarrassment for some women. There is no need to feel that way because milk ejection is natural. Your partner may feel jealous, and think your mind is on feeding the baby rather than on making love to him. (We now know that is not the case; rather, your milk is released as a result of pleasure). If you are concerned that your breast milk may be released during sex, have some tissue or a towel near you to wipe up any milk.

During the early postnatal period, if the baby is being breastfed some women have reported a significant decrease in libido or a complete loss of interest in sex. Hormonal changes associated with breastfeeding cause low levels of oestrogen in the vagina. For some women, this may cause vaginal dryness and they may experience discomfort during intercourse. A water-based lubricant such as Senselle or K-Y Jelly may help to lubricate your vagina. On the other hand, some women experience heightened sexual feelings as a result of the mixture of hormones in their body.

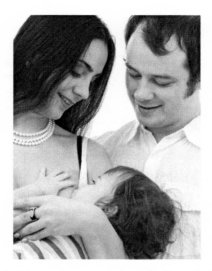

A dad showing interest in his baby breastfeeding

Support with breastfeeding.

Dr Pamela Jordan, who researched the effect of breastfeeding on men, said, "Just as the fathers are viewed as the primary support of the mother–baby relationship, the mother is the primary support to the father–baby relationship. Supporting the father during breastfeeding may help improve his, and consequently, the mother's, satisfaction with breastfeeding, the duration of breastfeeding and adaptation of both parents to parenthood."

It is important to get the dad involved. When he supports and encourages breastfeeding, you will be more interested in breastfeeding. You will be more successful and you will tend to breastfeed for longer – both of which will benefit your baby.

> *Did you know?*
>
> *Breastfeeding can use up to 500 calories a day, so if you breastfeed you can get your figure back quicker.*

Tips to consider when reclaiming your sex life:

- Seek help from the midwife, sex therapist or doctors if resuming sex becomes a major issue;
- If sex becomes painful, discuss this with your doctor. If necessary, he or she may prescribe medication to lessen pain and tenderness;
- Avoid feeling guilty if you don't feel ready to make love;
- When you are ready to have sex, take it slowly and do not forget to use contraception;
- Give signals that you are ready for sex. It can be as blatant as taking his hands and placing it on your breast or inside your pants. You can also provoke him by exposing certain parts of your body that you know he cannot resist;
- Keep your expectations in check: you may not reach orgasm on the first attempt, but remember it is a good start;
- Loosen up by massaging each other, showering together, or anything else that can help you to unwind and relax;
- Maintain intimacy in other ways if you are not ready for intercourse;
- You may temporarily experience dryness in the vagina due to hormonal changes after the birth. Use water-based

vaginal lubricant like K-Y Jelly or Senselle (the new name is Sensilube, a pure, greaseless, transparent, water-soluble and non-irritating lubricant) for intercourse. Avoid the use of petroleum jelly because it is oil based and may lead to infection;

- Side-to-side or the woman-on-top positions allow more control of depth of penetration and put less pressure on a sore perineum. Explore to find what works best for you;
- Be open with each other and talk things through;
- Talking to close friends who have had babies can help.

CHAPTER 7

Enhancing and maintaining your relationship through communication

The transition to parenthood is one of the most challenging milestones in a relationship. The birth of your baby can bring you together or push you apart. When some couples are faced with problems in their relationship, they believe having a baby will help bring them together and resolve their differences. This is a big mistake. The increased responsibilities that a new baby brings may be a source of stress on your relationship, and this could cause you to drift apart even more if your relationship is already rocky. Most couples ultimately discover that parenthood brings a whole new dimension to their relationship, one that enhances their intimacy and strengthens their bonding.

Job ad for new parents

> *Situation vacant: Mum/Dad*
> *Hours: 24 hours a day, 7 days a week, and on-call*
> *Annual leave: None*
> *Salary: None*
> *Contract: Commitment for life*
> *Benefits: Rewarding*

You may see yourself as more of a mother to your newborn than as a lover to your partner. The intimacy between mother and baby could pose a threat to a partner who may have previously enjoyed unrivalled intimacy and attention from you. The quality of your relationship can strongly influence the quality of your sexual experience. Trust and love play key roles in keeping sex and romance alive. The more affectionate the relationship, the better the companionship between you. Mutual affection brings about a deeper feeling of peace, security and comfort in the souls of the partners and any other children. To keep the fires lit, even if sex is not on the menu, try foreplay for a while and see how you feel.

To achieve a strong, healthy relationship, you have to work at it continuously. Steve and Shaaron Biddulph, the authors of *The Secret of Happy Parents*, have suggested ways to keep romantic. You need to set the scene and cultivate the place and space together. Things like colours, fabrics and shaded lighting can enhance your pleasure and stimulate your senses.

- Avoid putting clutter, such as books or clothing, on your bed;
- Make the bedroom tidy and relaxing for lovemaking;

- Don't use the bed for discussing your finances or renovation plans;
- Vary the location for lovemaking; you can make love on the floor in the lounge, on the sofa, or in the conservatory.

Keep talking

It is healthy to talk and listen to each other during this new adventure of taking care of a newborn baby. Take the opportunity to open your communication channels even more as you are both celebrating the new arrival. Many of us assume that our partners can read our minds. Opening up to each other about sexual matters will bring you closer to each other. Tell your partner about your expectations and needs with clarity to avoid misunderstanding.

Cherish each other's support

Have mutual respect for each other. Caring for a new baby is a big learning curve. Despite all the information from books, healthcare professionals and experiences shared by friends and family, you will still find a lot of unanswered questions when your baby arrives. For example, there are times when your baby will cry and nothing will seem to stop the tears. It can make you feel frustrated and helpless. Try to talk to each other rather than shouting, even when there is a misunderstanding.

Take care of yourselves

As your daily routine has changed dramatically, it is very easy to neglect yourself. Find time to pamper yourself and ensure you take care of your health. Looking good will help make you feel good. It is easy to let yourselves go when you are used to each other, especially when you are tired and stressed and caring for a newborn.

Let love and sex take their natural course

You may feel the need to resume sexual intercourse soon after delivery to please your partner, especially if you did not have much sex during pregnancy. There is no need to feel guilty or be under pressure to resume sexual intercourse. You have to feel ready physically and mentally to enjoy sex. If he says he feels neglected emotionally, do not ignore it. Tell him you understand and remind him that you are now also a mother, not just his partner. If you are not ready, you can both express your love in different ways to feel close. Kind gestures such as surprising each other with little presents – or simply making tea for each other – can make a difference.

Resolve problems immediately

Family members are usually helpful when the newborn arrives, but sometimes it can feel as if you're being taken over. They may want to do things that your partner may not be happy with. Do not overlook this and hope things will work out automatically. A build up of tension and anger can affect your love life. It can help everyone if you explain that there are some decisions that only you and your partner can make and that you know they will understand this need.

Connect with each other

Newborn babies need love, care and attention round the clock. Either of you can feel pushed away as the baby becomes the centre of attention. Playing your mothering role rather than that of a lover can make your partner feel neglected. Your partner may also unconsciously give most of his attention to the baby and very little to you. Though it may be difficult at first, arrange for a babysitter, so that you can plan simple but enjoyable activities together – even if it is just taking a walk, going out to eat, or having a picnic.

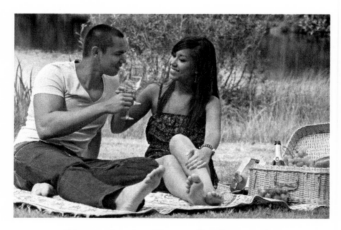

New parents spending quality time together

Give each other space

As much as it is important to spend quality time together, it is equally important to give each other a chance to have some alone time. Being in each other's space all the time can stifle the relationship. It is all about getting the balance right. Your partner can take care of the baby to give you some time to visit your friends, go to the hair salon, rest, or do some shopping. You might reciprocate so that he can watch football with his friends another time.

Some dads may be scared to be left alone at home to take care of the baby because the mum does not trust that he will "cope". When you treat a man as if he is inept, he will begin to feel inept. Let him feel that caring for a baby is part of his natural role as a father. Learn the skills of caring for a new baby *together*. Let him learn baby massage so that Daddy and baby can bond. Encourage your partner to change the baby's nappies, feed and bathe the baby even when you are around, so that these tasks become second nature when you are not around.

Save energy

When lovemaking is often the last event of the day, it can be a tug of war between sleep and stimulation.

- Ask for help from friends and family if you feel that the workload is becoming overwhelming;
- Prioritise and do the most important things first;
- Have an afternoon nap when your baby is sleeping;
- Put the kids to bed early;
- Go to bed early yourself to conserve more energy.

Women generally connect sex with the emotional aspect of the relationship. Women want a sense of connection, and for them intimacy starts well before sex is initiated. Men are more prone to visual stimulation and can respond very quickly. Be ready for the unexpected, and welcome his spontaneity.

We have learned that some of the factors which may dampen our sexual fire are: tiredness, hurt feelings, negative body image and rejection. Working with your partner will make you feel supported and loved. You will respond better and have more pleasure when you are making love because you are not exhausted from caring for the new baby and other housework. If there are any unresolved issues, taking the step to have an open and honest talk with your partner can help iron things out.

My work on this book has given me new insights into sex and childbirth. Through discussions with other midwives, obstetricians, parents and friends I have come to have a better understanding of how childbirth may affect perceptions of self, and sexual relationships. Above all, I hope this information will help to bring more harmony and awareness into your relationship during this life-changing experience of childbirth. Even when there are physical limitations to sex, you can still show love and affection and respect each other. Open and honest communication is the key to achieving a sexually fulfilling relationship following childbirth.

Glossary

Acetone/ketone: A chemical that is formed when the body uses fat instead of glucose (sugar) for energy. The formation of acetone means that cells lack insulin or cannot effectively use available insulin to burn glucose for energy. Acetone passes through the body into the urine as ketone bodies.

Anaesthetic: A substance that causes lack of feeling or awareness. A local anaesthetic causes loss of feeling in a certain part of the body. A general anaesthetic puts the person to sleep.

Body Image: The awareness and perception of your body in relation to both appearance and function.

Cervix (or neck of the womb): The lower, narrow portion of the uterus where it joins with the top end of the vagina.

Chloasma: Splashes of darkened skin that may appear on the forehead, nose and cheeks in a mask-like configuration on some pregnant women. It is found more in dark-skinned women.

Cholestasis: A rare complication in pregnancy that causes bile to build up in the bloodstream, causing itching, especially in the last trimester. It usually resolves after the birth.

Clitoris: The clitoris is the female sexual organ found where the labia minora, or inner lips, meet above the vaginal opening.

Colostrum: A special milk which is yellow to orange in colour and is thick and sticky. Colostrum is produced during pregnancy and continues through the early days of breastfeeding. It is low in fat and high in carbohydrates, protein and antibodies, to help keep your baby healthy. Colostrum is extremely easy to digest, and is therefore the perfect first food for your baby. It is low in volume (measurable in teaspoons rather than ounces), but high in concentrated nutrition for the newborn. Colostrum has a laxative effect on the baby, helping the baby pass the early stools, which aids in the excretion of dead red blood cells and helps prevent jaundice.

Douching: The word "douche" is French for "to wash". Douching is washing or cleaning out the vagina (also called the birth canal) with water or other mixtures of fluids. Douches were usually packaged mixes of water and vinegar, baking soda or iodine. Douching is not recommended anymore because it is known to introduce infection and reduce the good vaginal flora that women need.

Down's syndrome: A genetic disorder which is named after John Langdon Down, the doctor who first identified it. Down's syndrome affects your physical appearance as well as your ability to learn and develop mentally. It is a life-long condition that is present from birth. Down's syndrome occurs when a baby inherits an extra chromosome.

Episiotomy: An episiotomy is a surgical incision through the perineum made to enlarge the vagina and assist childbirth.

Fistula: A hole that develops between the vagina and the bladder and/or the rectum, resulting in steady leakage of urine and faeces. This is rare and usually occurs in women who are having difficulty in delivering and cannot receive medical care.

Lochia: A combination of blood, mucus and tissue that is discharged after birth. It is much like a period, beginning as a heavy flow and becoming lighter and brownish over time. All women have this discharge after birth, something midwives describe as "the weeping of the womb".

Labia: These are the folds of the vulva, and women have two sets: the inner (labia minora) and the outer (labia majora).

Oxytocin: A hormone made in the brain that plays a role in childbirth and lactation by causing muscles to contract in the womb and the mammary glands in the breast. Women having difficulty progressing in labour may be given the synthetic form of oxytocin, for strong and regular contraction.

Perineum: The area between the anus and vagina in the female, and the area between the anus and the scrotum in the male.

Prolactin: This is the main hormone involved in the formation and production of breast milk.

Placenta praevia: An obstetric complication in which the placenta is attached to the uterine wall close to or covering the cervix. It can sometimes occur in the later part of the first trimester, but is more usual during the second or third. It is a leading cause of a vaginal bleeding.

Spina bifida: It is a birth defect (a congenital malformation) in which there is a bony defect in the vertebral column, so that part of the spinal cord, which is normally protected within the vertebral column, is exposed.

Varicose veins: Varicose veins are swollen and enlarged veins which are usually a blue or dark purple. They may also be lumpy, bulging or twisted in appearance, and can be painful. They usually appear on the legs, but can sometimes appear on the vulva during pregnancy.

Vulva: The vulva is the external genital organs of the female.

References

1. Beckmann, M.M., Garrett, A.J. (2006) Antenatal perineal massage for reducing perineal trauma. Cochrane Database of Systematic Reviews. CD005123.

2. Biddulph, S., Biddulph, S. (2004) *The Secret of Happy Parents: How to stay in love as a couple and true to yourself.* Thorsons, London.

3. Health Promotion England (2006) *The Pregnancy Book: Your complete guide to pregnancy, childbirth and the first few weeks with a new baby.* HPE, London.

4. Calleja-Agius, J. (2008) Vaginal bleeding in the first trimester. *British Journal of Midwifery.* 16(10): 656-661.

5. De Angelis, B. (1990) *Secrets about Men every Woman Should Know.* Harper Collins, London.

6. Womenshealth.gov (2005) Douching: Frequently Asked Questions. US Department of Health and Human Services, Washington DC.

7. Houser, P.M. (2007) *Fathers-To-Be Handbook: A road map for the transition to fatherhood.* Creative Life Systems, Lamberhurst.

8. Kavanagh, J., Kelly, A.J., Thomas, J. (2001) Sexual intercourse for cervical ripening and induction of labour. Cochrane Database of Systematic Reviews. CD003093.

9. Mantle, J., Haslam, J., Barton, S. (2004) *Physiotherapy in Obstetrics and Gynaecology*. Second ed. Butterworth-Heinemann, Oxford.

10. Midwives Information and Resource Service (MIDIRS) (2008) Informed choice: Support in labour for women (leaflet). MIDIRS, Bristol.

11. Murkoff, H., Mazel, S. (2002) *What to Expect When You're Expecting*. Fourth ed. Workman Publishing, New York.

12. Physiotherapy Department (2009) Pelvic floor muscle exercises. Community Healthcare, Hounslow.

13. Polomeno, V. (2000) Sex and Pregnancy: A perinatal educator's guide. *Journal of Perinatal Education*. 9(4): 15-27.

14. Raven, J.H., Chen, Q., Tolhurst, R.J., Garner, P. (2007) Traditional beliefs and practices in the postpartum period in Fujian Province, China: a qualitative study. *BMC Pregnancy and Childbirth*. 7: 8.

15. Faculty of Sexual and Reproductive Healthcare (2009) *Postnatal Sexual and Reproductive Health*. FSRH, London.

16. Royal College of Psychiatrists (2007) Postnatal depression. RCPSYCH, London.

17. Sakornbut, E., Leeman, L., Fontaine, P. (2007) Late pregnancy bleeding. *American Family Physician*. 75(8): 1199-1206.

18. Stoppard, M. (2007) *New Pregnancy and Birth*. Dorling Kindersley, London.

19. Tan, P.C., Andi, A., Azmi, N., Noraihan, M.N. (2006) Effect of coitus at term on length of gestation, induction

of labour, and mode of delivery. *Obstetrics and Gynecology.* 108(1): 134-140.

20. Yettram, J. (2006) *Get Closer: Humps and Bumps – Sex during pregnancy and after giving birth.* National Childbirth Trust, London.

Websites

A low-lying placenta after 20 weeks (placenta praevia) www.rcog. org.uk women's health patients info.

Brott, A., www.mrdad.com/qa/firstyear/breastfeeding.html. Husbands and Breastfeeding.

Jones, C., www.birthingnaturally.net. The sexuality of childbirth.

Women's Health. www.womenshealth.gov/faq/douching.cfm. Douching.

Informed choice. www.infochoice.org

Birthing Naturally. www.birthingnaturally.net/cn/technique/ nipple.html Nipple stimulation for labour.

Schoenstadt, A., eMedTV. http://pregnancy.emedtv.com/ pregnancy-and-sex/sex-positions-during-pregnancy.html. Sex positions during pregnancy.

Online Muslim matrimonial. www.ezsoftech.com/omm/ handbook.asp. Islamic marriage handbook for young Muslims.

Hawaii Community College. http://www.hawcc.hawaii.edu/ nursing/RNChinese02.html. Chinese cultural beliefs related to pregnancy, birth and post-partum care.

Robin, H-C., www.robinhc.com/articles/communication/top-10-ways-enhance-your-relationship. Top 10 ways to enhance your relationship.

Resources and useful organisations

Household Companion Limited
Flat 6 Weston park
Weston
Hitchin
Hertfordshire
SG4 7BX
07768140044
www.householdcompanion.com
Specializes in delivering factual and fun sex education, as well as sex relationship therapy to
Parents (or parents- to- be) on how to sustain and maintain a fulfilling intimate relationship.

Relate
0300 100 1234
www.relate.org.uk
Relate offers relationship counselling for couples. They have centres throughout the country.

National Childbirth Trust
Alexandra House
London
W3 6NH
www.nct.org.uk
Organises antenatal classes and offers help after baby is born.

Association of Breastfeeding Mothers
PO Box 207
Bridgwater, Somerset
TA6 7YT
0870 401 7711
www.abm.me.uk
Offers 24-hour counselling services for mothers who are breastfeeding.

National Breastfeeding Helpline
03001000212
www.nationalbreastfeeding helpline.org.uk

The Multiple Births Foundation
Hammersmith House, Level 4
Queen Charlotte's and Chelsea Hospital
Du Cane Road
London
W12 0HS
0208 383 3519
www.multiplebirths.org.uk

Doula UK
PO Box 26678
London
N14 4WB
08714 333 103
www.doula.org.uk

Ecstatic Pregnancy and Birth
6 Court Lodge
Lamberhurst, Kent
TN3 8DU
01892 890 614
www.ecstaticbirth.com
An online childbirth education centre advocating a modern way of childbirth.

Association for Postnatal Illness
145 Dawes Road
Fulham
London
SW6 7EB
0207 386 0868
www.apni.org

MAMA: Meet a Mum Association
54 Lillington Road
Radstock, Avon
BA3 3NR
0845 120 3746
www.mama.co.uk

CRY-SIS Support group
BM CRY-Sis
0845122669
www.cry-sis.org.uk
Advice on babies who cry.

Family planning
British Pregnancy Advisory service (BPAS)
08703655050
www.bpas.org
Advice on contraception.

Institute for Complementary Medicine
www.icmedicine.co.uk

Lightning Source UK Ltd.
Milton Keynes UK
09 August 2010

158160UK00001B/4/P